more plants
on your plate

OVER 75 *fast and easy* **PLANT-FORWARD** RECIPES & MEAL PREP TIPS

BAILEY RHATIGAN

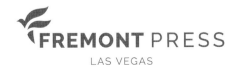

FREMONT PRESS

LAS VEGAS

First published in 2022 by Fremont Press

ISBN-13: 978-1-628604-43-6

The author is not a licensed practitioner, physician, or medical professional and offers no medical diagnoses, treatments, suggestions, or counseling. The information presented herein has not been evaluated by the U.S. Food and Drug Administration, and it is not intended to diagnose, treat, cure, or prevent any disease. Full medical clearance from a licensed physician should be obtained before beginning or modifying any diet, exercise, or lifestyle program, and physicians should be informed of all nutritional changes.

The author/owner claims no responsibility to any person or entity for any liability, loss, or damage caused or alleged to be caused directly or indirectly as a result of the use, application, or interpretation of the information presented herein.

Certain recipes in this book are sponsored by SILK and So Delicious, the author's favorite dairy alternative brands, along with RightRice. However, all opinions are the author's own.

Cover design by Charisse Reyes

Cover photo and lifestyle photos by Whitney Michelle Photo

Interior design by Charisse Reyes and Eli San Juan

Illustrations by Allan Santos

Recipe photos on pages 35, 43, 47, 53, 77, 99, 107, 115, 161, 167, 177, 179, 197, 199, 211, and 215 by Laura Scherb, Page & Plate Studios (www.pageandplate.com)

Printed in Canada
TC 0122

table of
contents

introduction • 4

My Story | 6

Why I Wrote This Book | 7

My Take on Plant-Forward | 8

Tips for Getting Started with Plant-Forward Eating | 9

Tips for Getting Started with Meal Prepping | 12

Pantry Staples and Grocery Shopping Strategy | 23

Easy Swaps for Food Allergies and Dietary Restrictions | 32

recipes • 34

1: Breakfast | 36

2: Meatless Mains | 66

3: Beef, Chicken & Turkey Recipes | 100

4: Date Night Recipes | 132

5: Salads & Sides | 150

6: Snacks | 168

7: Desserts | 188

8: Sauces & More | 210

index • 218

introduction

Hi! My name is Bailey, and I am so happy you've decided to incorporate more plants into your diet and purchased my cookbook to guide you.

This cookbook isn't geared specifically toward vegans or vegetarians. I've designed the recipes for people who want to eat less meat and add more plant foods to their meals. I follow only one mantra in my diet: **"How can I get more plants into this meal?"** Consequently, I offer a lot of fully plant-based meals and treats in this book, and some recipes have substitution options so that you can keep them fully plant-based if you wish. I also share some great meat-based recipes that include loads of veggies as well.

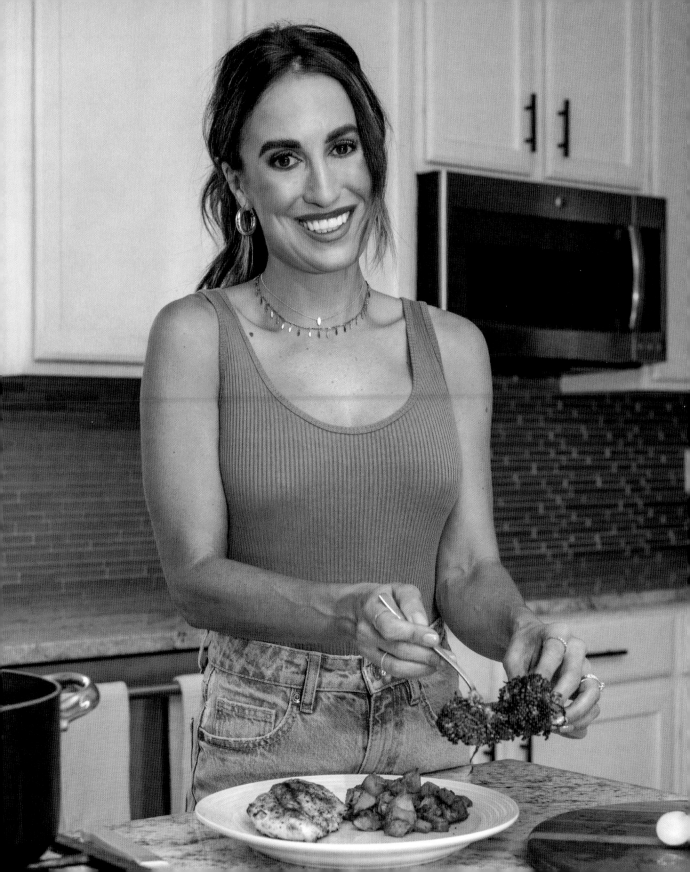

my story

My journey with plant-forward eating and meal prepping started about ten years ago. I was never a big meat eater, but I needed to keep meat in my diet due to low iron and vitamin B deficiencies. Those were issues I just couldn't correct by eating only plants, no matter how many supplements I tried. So I started to eat lean meat with my plant-based meals one to three times a week.

Some time later, I stumbled onto meal prepping. Matt, my soon-to-be-husband, started a job in the oil field; for two weeks nonstop, he was away in the middle of nowhere for work. Being health-conscious individuals, we knew he couldn't just load up on frozen meals and eat garbage. So we started prepping his meals the Sunday before he left for his work stint.

Our meal prep started out quite a mess. I think anyone who's just learning to meal prep can feel lost and overwhelmed like we did. The cheap plastic containers we used in the beginning were full of harmful chemicals, I'm sure, and for the first few weeks we relied heavily on spaghetti and lasagna. While Matt was away, I started experimenting with veggies and other plant foods, and I realized how amazing meals could taste if I added a few seasonings and varied my cooking methods. I remember adding coconut aminos to Brussels sprouts, broccoli, and mushrooms and being blown away by the flavors. Those first plant-forward meals were an achievement, but I'm happy to say that my recipes have come a long way since then.

Our meal prep Sundays took a major glow-up over time as we gained knowledge of what works and what doesn't and built our confidence. We purchased a big set of glass storage containers. We slowly started to figure out the quantities we needed for grocery shopping (so we could both have prepped meals while Matt was away) to avoid wasting food. We nailed down the routine, and we both enjoyed great meals throughout the week.

Matt's meals were the same as mine but were heavier on the meat. I added more veggies and plants to my portions both to stretch the meals further, saving us money, and because I find plant-heavy meals more appealing. It was the best of both worlds, and it continues to be to this day! Matt loves his meat, I love my veggies, and I try to marry the two in every meal throughout the week so we are both happy and getting the nutrients we need.

why I wrote this book

I created this cookbook to help people who want to eat more plants for the health benefits but don't want to drastically change their habits or eat boring food all week long. I also wanted to show people that meal prep doesn't have to be intimidating. It's not just for those who are looking to drop pounds quickly and compete in a bikini contest. It's not just for gym-goers who follow a very strict diet to maintain their physique. Meal prep is also for those of us who have busy schedules and don't want to succumb to takeout or salty packaged food every night, and for those who want to save money by shopping smart and cooking at home. Meal prep can be easy with the right setup and mindset, and I am confident this cookbook will help you see that little changes can impact your health and your wallet in a big way.

If you aren't looking to meal prep but just want to start eating more nutritious plant-forward meals, that's cool, too! This cookbook is a great place to start. Most of my recipes make two meals for two people or one meal for a family of four. I've even included treats and "date night meals" for you and your partner to enjoy on the weekends. Many of these dishes are best eaten fresh or take a little extra time to prepare, so they're perfect for when you want to stay in and treat yourself to a nice dinner.

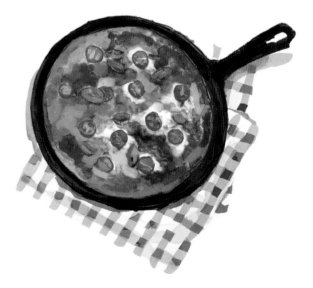

my take *on* plant-forward

Plant-forward is a style of cooking and eating that emphasizes plant foods but is not strictly limited to them. As I mentioned earlier, this book isn't only for vegans or vegetarians. You can still eat whatever you like; you'll simply be incorporating more plants into your meals as you eat a little less meat and dairy.

As a plant-forward eater, I still enjoy meat and dairy every week. Instead of having those foods at every meal, though, I may go three days of the week without cow's milk products or meat, and I eat smaller amounts than I used to on the other days. I feel my best eating this way, and you may notice that you also feel great with plant-forward eating! But hey, if you love meat, I suggest options for including meat in almost every recipe that doesn't already call for it.

If you want to be or already are a vegetarian, high-five! That's amazing. Most of my recipes have options for you. And if your diet is 100 percent plant-based (vegan), I have your back, too. When a recipe includes animal products, I suggest substitutions or other alterations to make the dish work within your diet.

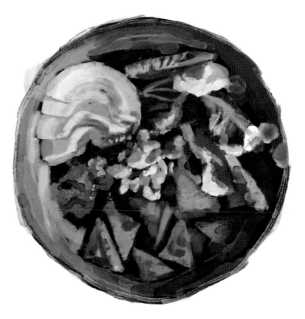

tips for getting started *with* plant-forward eating

If you're feeling unsure about how to get more plants on your plate, here are some things to consider.

Think about what your favorite leafy green is.
Is it kale or romaine lettuce? Or maybe it's spinach or mixed greens? Whatever green you like best, I want you to focus on that with a lot of these recipes. If there is a veggie you don't like, switch it out for one you enjoy. If I suggest kale but you despise it (hey, a lot of folks do; it's nothing to worry about!), you can substitute another leafy green, like spinach or romaine lettuce. If you dislike spinach and I call for it in a cooked dish, use mixed greens or kale instead. My primary goal is to help you find ways to eat more plants and be super excited about mealtime. I don't want you feeling deprived and forcing down veggies you don't like. I am all about customizing recipes to suit your palate.

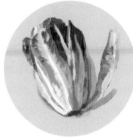

Think about what your favorite veggies are.
I'll be the first to admit that textures can really turn people off, so if you really don't care for a particular veggie, no problem. Think about your favorite vegetables. Do you dislike broccoli? Use another cruciferous veggie, like cauliflower or cabbage, instead. I call for a lot of zucchini, mushrooms, and broccoli in this cookbook because those vegetables are typically very affordable and offer great nutrition, but if you prefer bell peppers, cauliflower, and eggplant, great! Those substitutes will likely work just as well. Again, customize the recipes based on what you enjoy. We all have different opinions when it comes to veggies.

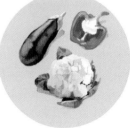

Get creative about adding veggies to foods you like.
Here are some suggestions to spark creativity for your future cooking endeavors:

Baked goods: Add ¼ cup or more of shredded zucchini or carrots to muffins and quick breads to boost the nutrients and get more veggies into your diet. Chances are you won't even taste the veggies you sneaked in, and most recipes will still turn out fine.

You can also use a chia or flax egg instead of a chicken egg in baked goods to cut down on animal products. Yes, baking is a science, and following a recipe as written is important, but I am confident that a chia or flax egg swap will work great the majority of the time. To make a chia or flax egg, just mix 1 tablespoon of chia or ground flax seeds with 2½ tablespoons of water and let it soak until a gel forms, 5 to 8 minutes.

Eggs: Mix chopped veggies into scrambled eggs—spinach, mushrooms, peppers, onions, you name it. The more veggies you add, the fewer eggs you need.

Meatballs and meatloaf: Chopped mushrooms take on a similar texture to ground meat, so they can easily be mixed into meatballs, meatloaf, and other dishes. You can also mix finely chopped zucchini with lean meat to keep it moist and use it to help stretch other meat dishes.

Roasted chicken: Always plan to roast several chopped veggies when you roast chicken. You can use hardy vegetables like Brussels sprouts, carrots, and parsnips in place of or in addition to potatoes.

Sauces, soups, and stews: If you are making a spaghetti sauce or any other style of sauce to pour over chicken, fish, or noodles, add handfuls of spinach or finely chop your favorite veggies to mix into the sauce! The same goes for soups and stews. I can assure you that no dish will be ruined by a little boost of veggies. Carrots go wonderfully in red sauces. You can blend them in or leave little chunks to give a sauce more texture. Spinach wilts nicely into just about any savory dish, and it is a great source of iron. You can also sneak all sorts of veggies into a meal by blending them up and making a chimichurri-style sauce (find my recipe on page 213).

Sort out your spice drawer.
Spices and seasonings are generally the stars of a recipe. They take meals from blah to YUM. My go-to dried seasonings include chili powder, chipotle powder, cumin, garlic powder, Italian seasoning, paprika, rosemary, and thyme, along with salt and pepper. I don't buy premade seasoning blends much because they tend to take up space in my

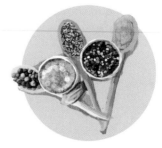

drawer without getting much use; they are more expensive and can easily be made at home as needed. But again, you can customize every recipe in this book. If you don't want to make your own easy taco seasoning and would rather use a packet, no problem. If you don't like thyme, you likely can leave it out without drastically changing the outcome of the recipe. I want you to feel confident that you can customize these recipes to fit your taste buds without ruining the dish.

Keep the ingredients simple and affordable.
I am all about easy meals. I don't call for obscure ingredients, such as truffles flown in from Europe, enoki mushrooms foraged from Asia, or Roquefort cheese crumbles. I promise you that I shop at the same kinds of grocery stores where you probably shop. I go to big-box stores and look for deals on fresh produce. I go for local farm-fresh veggies and fruits, and I also focus on seasonal items. All these recipes are attainable for anyone. If you live in the middle of nowhere and there is only a Walmart near you, this cookbook will work for you. If you live in a big city and are surrounded by Whole Foods Markets and independent natural food stores, this cookbook will work for you, too!

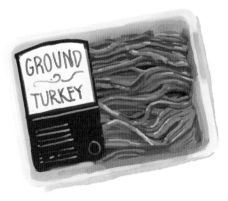

My personal checklist when it comes to selecting ingredients for my recipes includes these considerations:

- Is it easy to prepare?

- Is it nutrient-dense?

- Can I get it at any grocery store?

- Is it affordable?

As long as all of those boxes are checked, then I am happy to make the recipe available to you!

When I am meal prepping for the week, I buy smaller amounts of meat and use more veggies in place of the meat. For example, if I am making turkey tacos for the week for the two of us, I buy 1 pound of ground turkey—1 pound to last two people all week! I bulk up the recipe by adding a few chopped zucchinis and chopped mushrooms so that in every serving, we are getting less meat and more veggies versus all meat and no veggies.

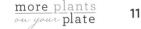

tips for getting started *with* meal prepping

You can meal prep most of the recipes in this book. I designed the recipes so that two people will get two to three days' worth of prepped meals. However, not everyone requires the same amount of food; you may find that you have plenty of food for more days or that you have enough for only a couple of days. Feel free to scale the recipes up or down to suit your appetite.

Here are some of my key strategies for meal prepping:

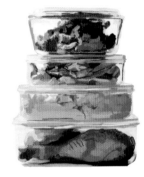

I like to do my shopping and meal prepping over the weekend so that I have meals ready to go for the workweek. Some people like to split up the prepping and cooking tasks over two days, with the second day falling midweek, so that they have fresher meals for the second half of the week, or to change things up and prevent meal boredom.

Choose recipes that use some of the same ingredients in different ways. This is the key to minimizing food waste and keeping meal prep simple. For example, the recipes for Turkey Veggie Tacos (page 130) and Zoodles with Artichoke Pesto & Mushrooms (page 72) both call for zucchini; if you have leftover mushrooms from the tacos, you can toss them into your zoodle dish! Or you can do a Cauliflower Hash (page 46) the same week you make Baked Spiced Cauliflower (page 151).

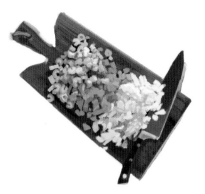

First, get the oven preheated and bring water to a boil if needed for the recipes you are meal prepping. While you're waiting, you can start chopping your veggies.

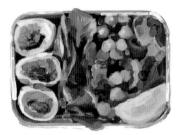

Cook your grains (rice, quinoa, and so on) in large batches and then portion them out.

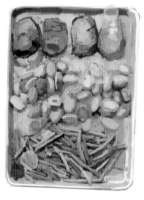

Get foods that need to cook longer into the oven first, and then take care of other tasks while those foods are baking.

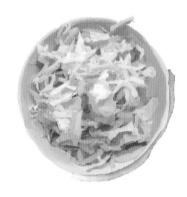

Any fresh ingredients that will not go into cooked dishes, such as toppings for tacos or burgers, can be prepped and stored in separate containers in the refrigerator and then added to the meal just before serving.

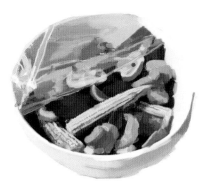

Look for opportunities to use up leftover veggies and greens from the fridge.

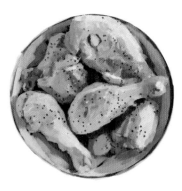

Remember that reheating causes foods to cook more, so be careful not to overcook foods like chicken when you are meal prepping.

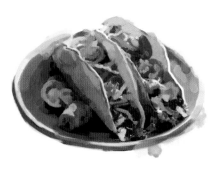

Mix and match prepped components to create whole new meals. For example, you could add leftovers from the Beef Spaghetti Squash with Tzatziki (page 128) to a breakfast hash to give it a unique flavor. Or you could take leftover fillings from any of the various taco recipes and make a quesadilla, salad, or rice bowl.

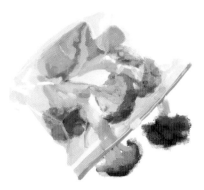

Take advantage of the freezer. You can freeze most of your leftovers in individual serving-size bags. When needed, pull one out of the freezer and defrost it in the refrigerator overnight, then heat it up the next day. Breakfast Burritos (page 54) work wonderfully! You can also freeze leftover raw veggies in airtight containers for later use.

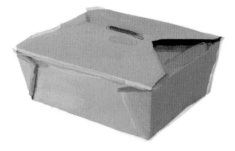

Allow for takeout and restaurant meals. Be realistic about how many prepped meals you'll need throughout the week so you don't end up making too many.

Essential Meal Prep Equipment

To prepare you for meal prepping and using this cookbook in general, I want to suggest a few items to help you execute these recipes with ease and a few items to purchase or have on hand for storing prepped meals and components.

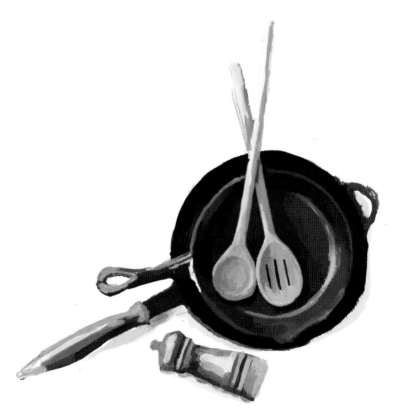

Cooking Items

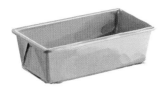

Loaf pans: I suggest having one loaf pan for meatloaf and other savory dishes and another for baked goods. I have noticed that my meat/savory pan gets slightly more beat up than my bread/dessert pan, which is why I like to have one for each purpose. To make the recipes in this book, you will need a 9 by 5-inch and a 8½ by 4½-inch loaf pan.

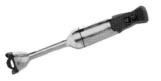

Food processor or high-powered blender: This appliance is very important for any chef or home cook; it can truly make or break a recipe! You want a standard-size one that works really well.

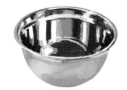

Immersion blender: This is a pretty inexpensive tool, and it's one of my favorites to use in the kitchen. An immersion blender makes the best dressings and sauces.

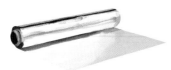

Mixing bowls: Every kitchen needs a great set of mixing bowls. You can find a nice set at any big box store, and they can fit inside each other to save cabinet space.

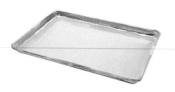

Parchment paper and aluminum foil: I use one or both every time I bake or cook a meal. Parchment paper prevents foods from sticking to your pans and makes cleanup much easier.

Rimmed baking sheets and cookie sheets: You will want two large baking sheets with an edge on all four sides, also known as sheet pans. Having at least two on hand will come in handy for the recipes in this book! In addition, make sure you have a couple of flat baking sheets, also called cookie sheets, to bake cookies and pizza.

Storage Items

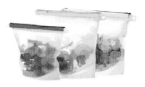

Food storage bags: Resealable plastic bags or freezer-friendly reusable bags such as Stasher bags are good for storing foods like meatballs, cookies, and leftover veggies, so stock up.

Glass food storage containers: I prefer glass storage containers for my prepped meals because glass lasts longer and is safer for cooling and reheating food. If you have only plastic containers, just check to make sure they are free of BPA, particularly when using the containers to microwave or freeze food. I suggest you have a few 2-cup containers and a few 1-quart containers, but you'll need some bigger and smaller sizes as well. I have four 2-quart containers and four 3-quart containers; these are the sizes I use most often for leftovers. You can find a lot of great sets of glass containers in various sizes on Amazon.com or at large chain stores like Target and Walmart. We've had our containers for six years, and they've been totally worth the investment.

Storing and Reheating Prepped Meals and Components

Storing food doesn't need to be complicated; it just takes some planning. If you want to make a few meals for the week ahead and you plan to eat them within 5 days, you will want to store the food in the refrigerator.

Pro tip: If you are approaching the 4-day mark and you don't think you're going to have the opportunity to eat the meal, get it into the freezer ASAP. Then you will have a month or more to warm it up and enjoy it.

If you are thinking long term and want to meal plan at the beginning of the month for the coming weeks, or if you just want to make a few meals to have on hand in the freezer for when life gets extra busy, I suggest you freeze the meals as soon as they have fully cooled.

The chart on the following pages gives you some guidelines for food storage.

FOOD	TYPE	Refrigerator (40°F or below)	Freezer (0°F or below)
Salad	Egg, chicken, ham, tuna, and macaroni salads	3 to 4 days	Does not freeze well
Hot dogs	Opened package	1 week	1 to 2 months
	Unopened package	2 weeks	1 to 2 months
Lunchmeat	Opened package or deli sliced	3 to 5 days	1 to 2 months
	Unopened package	2 weeks	1 to 2 months
Bacon and sausage	Bacon	1 week	1 month
	Sausage, raw, from chicken, turkey, pork, or beef	1 to 2 days	1 to 2 months
	Sausage, fully cooked, from chicken, turkey, pork, or beef	1 week	1 to 2 months
	Sausage, purchased frozen	After cooking, 3 to 4 days	1 to 2 months from date of purchase
Ground meats and ground poultry	Ground beef, turkey, chicken, other poultry, veal, pork, lamb, and mixtures of them	1 to 2 days	3 to 4 months
Fresh beef, veal, lamb, and pork	Steaks, chops, or roasts	3 to 5 days	4 to 12 months

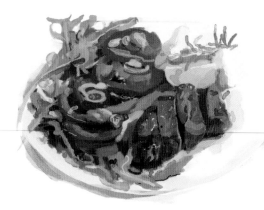

FOOD	TYPE	Refrigerator (40°F or below)	Freezer (0°F or below)
Ham	Fresh, uncured, uncooked	3 to 5 days	6 months
	Fresh, uncured, cooked	3 to 4 days	3 to 4 months
	Wet-cured, uncooked	5 to 7 days or "use by" date	3 to 4 months
	Fully cooked, vacuum-sealed at plant, unopened	2 weeks or "use by" date	1 to 2 months
	Cooked, store-wrapped, whole	1 week	1 to 2 months
	Cooked, store-wrapped, slices, half, or spiral cut	3 to 5 days	1 to 2 months
	Country ham, cooked	1 week	1 month
	Dry-cured, such as prosciutto, Parma, or Serrano	2 to 3 months	1 month
Fresh poultry	Chicken or turkey, whole	1 to 2 days	1 year
	Chicken or turkey, pieces	1 to 2 days	9 months
Fin fish	Fatty fish (bluefish, catfish, mackerel, mullet, salmon, tuna, etc.)	1 to 3 days	2 to 3 months
	Lean fish (cod, flounder, haddock, halibut, sole, etc.)		6 to 8 months
	Lean fish (pollock, ocean perch, rockfish, sea trout)		4 to 8 months

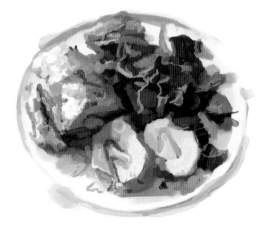

FOOD	TYPE	Refrigerator (40°F or below)	Freezer (0°F or below)
Shellfish	Shrimp, crayfish	3 to 5 days	6 to 18 months
	Shucked clams, mussels, oysters, and scallops	3 to 10 days	3 to 4 months
Eggs	Raw eggs in shell	3 to 5 weeks	Do not freeze in shell. Beat yolks and whites together, then freeze
	Raw egg whites and yolks	2 to 4 days	12 months *Note:* Yolks do not freeze well
	Hard-cooked eggs	1 week	Do not freeze
	Egg substitutes, liquid, unopened	1 week	Do not freeze
	Egg substitutes, liquid, opened	3 days	Do not freeze
	Egg substitutes, frozen, unopened	After thawing, 1 week, or refer to "use by" date	12 months
	Egg substitutes, frozen, opened	After thawing, 3 to 4 days, or refer to "use by" date	Do not freeze
	Casseroles with eggs	After baking, 3 to 4 days	After baking, 2 to 3 months
	Pies: pumpkin or pecan	After baking, 3 to 4 days	After baking, 1 to 2 months
	Pies: custard and chiffon	After baking, 3 to 4 days	Do not freeze
	Quiche with filling	After baking, 3 to 5 days	After baking, 2 to 3 months
Soups and stews	Vegetable or meat added	3 to 4 days	2 to 3 months

FOOD	TYPE	Refrigerator (40°F or below)	Freezer (0°F or below)
Leftovers	Cooked meat or poultry	3 to 4 days	2 to 6 months
	Chicken nuggets or patties	3 to 4 days	1 to 3 months
	Pizza	3 to 4 days	1 to 2 months

Source: https://www.foodsafety.gov/food-safety-charts/cold-food-storage-charts

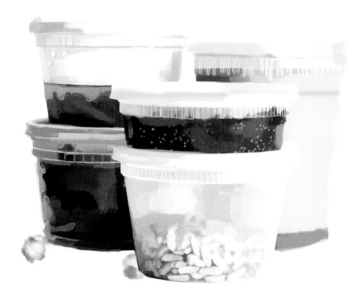

Reheating Best Practices

If you are reheating meat, bread, or cheese from the freezer, it should be defrosted before being reheated in a skillet or in the oven. You can certainly use the microwave as well; burritos, eggs, and rice- or quinoa-based dishes are great reheated in the microwave. The only thing I do not like to reheat in the microwave is cooked chicken; I prefer to use the oven, an air fryer, or a skillet for chicken. If you are reheating meatballs or meatloaf, I suggest defrosting it a bit if frozen and reheating in the microwave covered with a damp paper towel for 3 to 4 minutes, or you can reheat meatballs in sauce for 5 to 8 minutes on the stovetop.

If you are reheating frozen veggies, you can toss them right into a saucepan with a spritz of oil; this should keep them from getting soggy.

Breads can be reheated in an air fryer or in the oven on a low heat setting; you can also reheat them in the microwave on low for 30 to 90 seconds. Cookies can be eaten right out of the freezer or be defrosted for a few minutes. Desserts are great to store in the freezer. Keeping them frozen will help with self-control, and you'll have something a bit healthier on hand when you get a sweet tooth! I also like to freeze batches of some of my dessert recipes (like my Almond Lemon Cookies on page 206) for when we have unexpected company. I can pull the treats out of the freezer prior to my guests' arrival and have a great homemade dessert ready to serve.

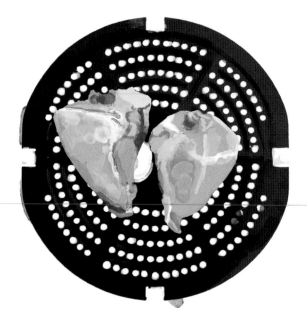

pantry staples *and* grocery shopping strategy

Having a well-stocked pantry is important for cooking and meal prepping success. In this section, I list the pantry items I always keep on hand to ensure I have what I need to make healthy meals. I also explain what you can do to eat as many plants as possible.

To get more plants on your plate, you need a grocery shopping strategy for fresh foods. Here, I'll explain which vegetables and fruits I buy on each of my grocery trips. Make sure to keep your favorite veggies on hand to sneak into your cooking. Your favorites should become staples on your grocery list. For me, those staple items are mushrooms, spinach, zucchini, and broccoli or cauliflower.

Make a list before going to the grocery store. I write down my planned meals in the upper-right corner, and then I list all the ingredients I need to make those meals, grouped according to the layout of the store (all the produce together, all the dairy items together, and so on). Having the meals written on the list helps me visualize what I'm planning to make, and this method might work for you, too. Of course, the list is just a starting point; you might get inspired to add some different veggies to the meal you have planned once you get to the produce aisles and see what looks best that week!

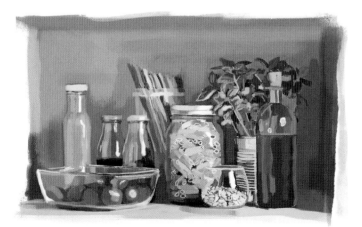

Dried Herbs and Spices

As I mentioned earlier, there are a handful of dried herbs and spices that I always have on hand. The majority of my recipes call for one or more of these go-to seasonings:

- Black peppercorns
- Chili powder
- Chipotle powder
- Garlic powder
- Ground cinnamon
- Ground cumin
- Ground dried oregano

- Ground dried rosemary
- Ground dried thyme
- Italian seasoning
- Marjoram
- Onion powder
- Paprika

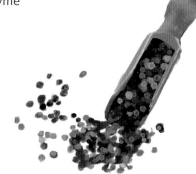

When using leafy dried herbs like Italian seasoning, be sure to crush them a bit between your fingertips or in your hand. This helps to "wake up" the flavor. I learned this trick on a PBS cooking show when I was a teenager, and it has stuck with me ever since.

Fresh Herbs

Fresh herbs make your meals look more appealing and taste even more fantastic than when you use dried herbs. I only buy fresh herbs as needed at the beginning of each week. Here are some herbs that I commonly use:

- Basil
- Cilantro
- Dill
- Parsley (curly or flat-leaf)
- Rosemary

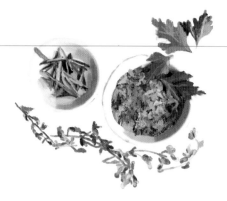

To keep herbs as fresh as possible, I suggest submerging them in a big bowl of water and ice cubes and keeping it in your refrigerator. Trust me, this will prolong their life and keep them from wilting. You can periodically add ice cubes to the bowl to continue preserving the herbs.

Fruits and Vegetables

- **Apples:** Apples keep for quite some time in the refrigerator, and they are great in oatmeal or baked up for dessert or a snack.

- **Avocados:** I typically buy avocados when they are very hard and not ripe. I buy four or five at a time because I love them! When I get home, I leave them on the counter to soften just a little and then put them in the refrigerator. They soften slowly in the fridge; five avocados typically last me about two weeks. I just pull out the softest one when I'm ready to use it. If you haven't tried storing your avocados in the refrigerator, you are missing out on a handy trick to slow the ripening!

- **Bananas:** Bananas are always great for baking, and they work nicely for topping oats, pancakes, or waffles. I also like them as a pre- or post-workout snack. If you find that you end up with a lot of brown spotty bananas, cut them into coins, place them in a resealable plastic bag, and store them in the freezer for up to 4 months for use in smoothies, baked goods, and more.

- **Blueberries:** Blueberries are my must-have fruit. I bake with them, snack on them, and top my oatmeal with them. They are in my cart every week.

- **Broccoli:** I always have 1 to 2 pounds in my refrigerator. I chop it all up when I get home, leave in the bag I bought it in, and use it in recipes as well as in sides for extra meals, like spontaneous lunches or date night dinners. For example, if we decide to have grilled chicken in the middle of the week, I have broccoli ready to steam and season.

- **Mushrooms:** I often grab a pack of sliced mushrooms and add them to dishes that call for ground turkey or beef. Chopped mushrooms add texture and help stretch a meal further so you can use less meat.

- **Onions and garlic:** If you want to make insanely good food that's full of flavor, you will want to stock up on onions and garlic. No more minced garlic in the jar! Fresh garlic offers so much more flavor—you may be surprised by how much of a difference there is. Once you get your garlic mincing technique down, you will see that using fresh garlic doesn't take as much effort as you once thought.

- **Spinach:** A bag of spinach makes its way into my cart every week. Even when it gets wilty, I chop it up and microwave it with leftovers or add it to soups, roasted or sautéed veggies, or sauces. It is such an easy green to incorporate into your diet. You can also store spinach in the freezer! Frozen spinach is great for adding to smoothies or just about any recipe that calls for spinach. It doesn't get soggy when frozen.

- **Sweet potatoes:** I love sweet potatoes with many meals. I also make sweet potato fries on Sunday to have on hand for snacks or lunch/dinner sides (see page 162 for the recipe). The leftovers often make it onto my salads as well. You can use regular potatoes instead of sweet potatoes in any of my recipes, but sweet potatoes offer a bit more nutrition.

- **Zucchini:** As I said before, I use a lot of zucchini. Zucchini is always affordable and abundant, and it's a great plant filler for recipes.

What are your favorite fruits and veggies? Think about what you like, and try to develop a habit of keeping your kitchen stocked with them so that you eat plenty of them. But don't shy away from trying new ones, too!

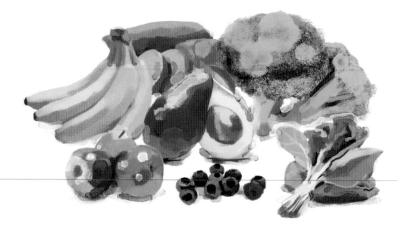

Eggs, Egg Alternatives, Dairy, and Dairy Alternatives

Every household should be stocked up on these items. I use them for baking and to add a creamy texture or flavorful sauce to savory dishes. Of course, if you are not eating eggs and/or dairy, you are welcome to use plant-based alternatives, which usually work just as well in cooking and baking.

- **Eggs:** I love eggs, and I eat them often. They make a great snack!

- **Egg alternatives:** If you are avoiding eggs, be sure to stock up on egg replacement powder, chia seeds, and/or ground flax seeds to use in place of eggs in baked goods.

- **Plant-based milk alternatives or dairy milk:** I try to minimize my dairy intake, so a lot of my recipes call for plant-based milk alternatives. My favorites are SILK unsweetened almond milk and So Delicious unsweetened coconut milk. If you prefer dairy milk, you can substitute that in any of my recipes.

- **So Delicious CocoWhip:** This product is sold at most natural food stores in the freezer section, and it is my favorite sweet treat from the fridge or freezer. It is naturally very low in sugar per serving, and because it is plant-based, it's a great alternative to regular whipped cream or ice cream. I've included a few recipes that call for this whipped treat.

- **So Delicious Original coconut milk creamer:** I buy this for use in recipes that need a nondairy alternative to heavy cream, which is thicker than milk. If you consume dairy, you may substitute heavy cream in any of my recipes that call for coconut milk creamer.

- **Yogurt, dairy and/or plant-based:** Unsweetened Greek yogurt is a great option to stock in the fridge. I always buy a tub of So Delicious unsweetened coconut yogurt, too. It works well in recipes that call for dairy yogurt, it is a delicious snack, and you can make wonderful sauces and dressings with it.

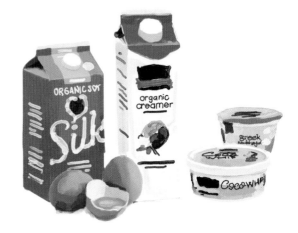

Pantry Items and Condiments

You can't make a great meal without pantry items or condiments! Several of the recipes in this book call for the following items, which I keep stocked year-round and use in almost all recipes, or at least often enough to have an arsenal of them on hand.

- Avocado oil: If you don't like olive oil or can't find a neutral-tasting brand, avocado oil is a great alternative. Avocado oil is a little more expensive than olive oil, but it is very mild and works great for high-heat cooking, such as roasting vegetables.

- Canned beans: I always have a few cans of beans in my pantry. They can be added to just about any lunch or dinner. I often add a can of beans to a dish to make it go further while still being filling.

- Chia seeds: I use chia seeds in oatmeal and chia puddings and also as an egg replacer in a few recipes (see page 10).

- Coconut aminos/liquid aminos: Coconut aminos and liquid aminos are great alternatives to soy sauce but have a lighter flavor. You typically find these products in the same aisle where the soy sauce is located. If you prefer soy sauce, you can use it in place of coconut aminos in any recipe. Tamari also works wonderfully; it is a bit richer in flavor than the other products mentioned above.

- Olive oil: I use two types of olive oil. The first is extra-virgin olive oil, which has a strong taste. I use it for moderate-heat cooking and as a finishing oil, drizzling it over salads or toasts for a pop of flavor—a little goes a LONG WAY. The other is an olive oil that's light in color and has a neutral flavor. Look for words like "mild," "light," and "neutral" on the labels in the oil aisle. I often buy Bertolli brand olive oil; they make an olive oil that says "extra light tasting" on the label. You can also use avocado oil in place of olive oil in any recipe.

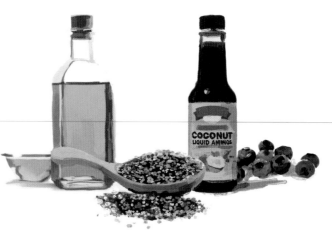

- **Miso paste:** Miso paste gives foods a salty umami flavor. I use it a lot when I make my own dressings. It's typically found in the international foods aisle.

- **Old-fashioned oats:** I usually buy three of the big 2-pound containers of oats to stock up for a month. I use oats in several recipes, and we eat a lot of overnight oats and stovetop oats throughout the week. You can use oats to make gluten-free oat flour, granola (see page 56), baked goods, and more. I also often use oats in place of breadcrumbs.

- **Raw nuts:** Almonds, cashews, and walnuts are my go-to nuts. I always stay stocked up on these three for recipes and quick healthy snacks. Just be sure to watch your portions—if you're like me, you probably can get out of control with nuts.

- **RightRice:** This rice is made from veggies and offers a lot of protein for a plant-based/vegan product. I order mine on Amazon, but a lot of grocery stores sell it. A few of my recipes call for this specific brand. It is so quick to whip up for a side, and it adds more servings of plants to any meal. If you prefer, you can use another type of rice, such as white or brown rice (regular or instant) or even cauliflower rice.

- **Salsa:** When I'm feeling lazy or I have random leftovers in the fridge, I use salsa as a dressing. I also use it on eggs and to spruce up leftover tacos. Salsa has a lot of veggies in it, and it's available in many flavor varieties, so you can easily spruce up meals with it or change up a classic meal by adding a different flavor of salsa. I always grab a jar or two when I shop.

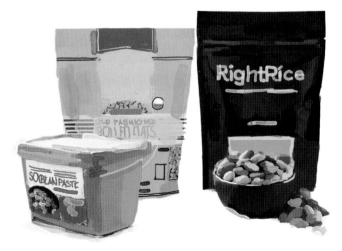

Snacks

Having snacks like these on hand throughout the week will help you make healthy choices when you find yourself hungry between meals:

- **Easy-to-eat veggies:** Carrots, cucumbers, and mini sweet peppers are crunchy snacks that make healthy vehicles for dip. I often sprinkle a tiny bit of salt on cucumbers to help curb a salty-savory chip craving. Mini peppers are perfect for stuffing with cheese or hummus for a plant-y snack. Precut broccoli and cauliflower florets are also great for dipping in leftover pesto (page 72), garlic sauce (page 216), and more.

- **High-protein yogurt or yogurt alternatives:** This is a super satisfying snack! When you purchase yogurt or yogurt alternatives, be sure to look at the sugar and protein contents. Low sugar and high protein is the goal when it comes to yogurt.

- **Homemade granola:** I make this throughout the year (see my recipe on page 56) and always try to have a container of it in my pantry.

- **Hummus:** The homemade hummus on page 178 is wonderful, but for busy weeks, I recommend buying premade hummus for a healthy plant-based snack. We eat hummus weekly with chopped raw veggies or leftover roasted veggies. We also use it on sandwiches and dip leftover tortillas in it.

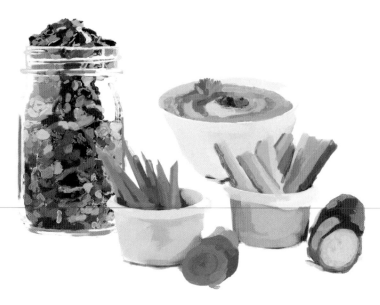

- **Lesser Evil Clean Snacks:** I buy these vegan puffs from Amazon.com, and they are a great alternative to greasy chips or cheese puffs. They are made from plants and come in several flavors. I prefer the "No Cheese Cheesiness" Paleo Puffs, Himalayan Pink Salt Paleo Puffs, and Vegan Ranch Veggie Sticks. The company also makes healthy plant-based popcorn.

- **Peanut butter/nut butter:** You can use it to make my Vegan Peanut Butter Cookies (page 202), add it to smoothies, dip apples in it, and so much more. Always be sure you are stocked up on peanut butter or the nut butters you like best!

- **Popcorn:** Popcorn has fiber and antioxidants, which make it a great crunchy snack. When purchasing prepopped popcorn, be mindful of the brand. You want a clean popcorn with low fat and sugar contents. I prefer Lesser Evil or Smart Pop.

- **Turkey jerky:** I always have Chomps turkey sticks or Costco's bulk turkey jerky in my pantry for a high-protein, low-fat snack. I also carry a few turkey sticks in my purse for instant energy when I am running errands or traveling.

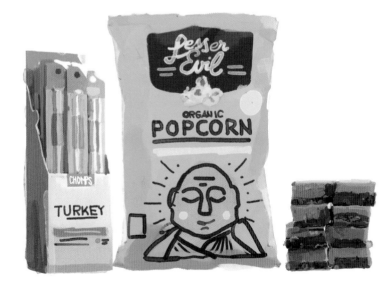

easy swaps for food allergies *and* dietary restrictions

Some people have to be selective about what they eat because of food allergies and other dietary restrictions, so I've listed some easy swaps you can make as you work through the recipes in this cookbook. Aside from these general swaps, I offer some meat/meatless/nondairy suggestions in the recipes where those substitutions are applicable. The following suggestions should really help you if you have a question in the back of your mind:

- **All-purpose flour:** Gluten-free 1:1 baking flour

- **Butter:** Vegan butter (such as Earth Balance or margarine), coconut oil, or olive oil

- **Cheese:** Plant-based cheese, goat cheese, Manchego, or fresh mozzarella (I find that my body tolerates sheep, goat, and European cheeses better than cow's milk cheeses made in the US.)

- **Chicken breast:** Portobello mushrooms, tofu, or tempeh

- **Eggs:** Chia egg, flax egg, or egg replacement powder (see page 10)

- **Ground turkey or chicken:** Lentils, tempeh, or chopped mushrooms

- **Peanut butter:** Almond butter, cashew butter, or sunflower seed butter

- **Sour cream:** Vegan sour cream (such as Tofutti brand), plain Greek yogurt, or blended soft tofu

- **Yogurt:** Coconut yogurt (such as So Delicious brand), almond yogurt, cashew yogurt, or sour cream (if you don't like yogurt)

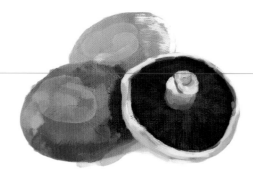

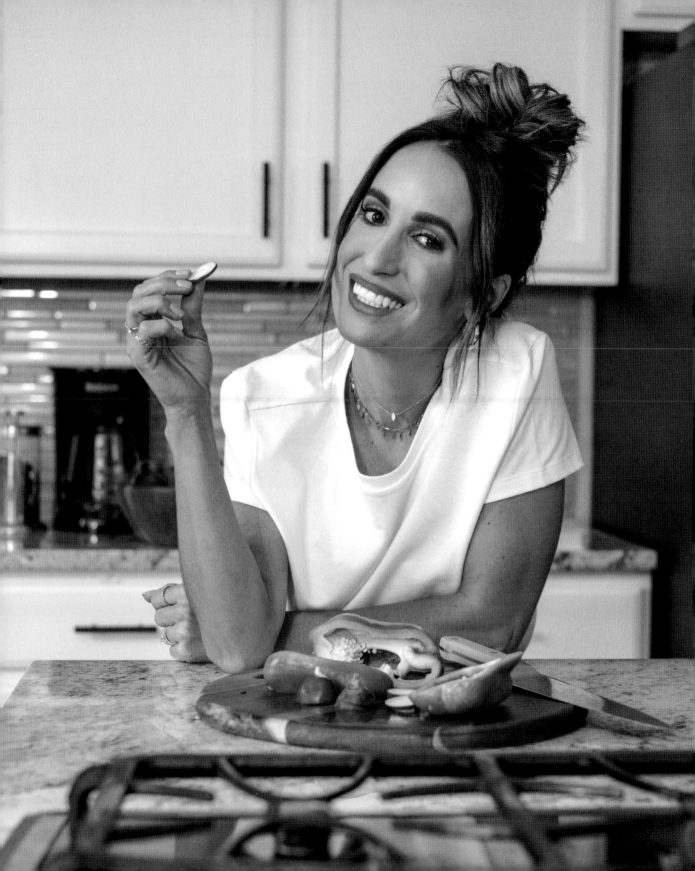

recipes

I said earlier that eating well is a way of respecting yourself. An inextricable part of eating well is cooking. Life can get pretty busy, but just as movement, self-care, and regular dentist appointments are priorities, cooking needs to factor in there, too. I'm not guilt-tripping you. If you've been resistant to cooking, I get it: No one taught you how, or you don't think you're any good. You work crazy hours and/or have a hectic household. Kids, pets, schedules, life. The chaos around us will always be there. Still, I urge you to spend time in the kitchen. The key to changing your eating habits begins with truly connecting with the food you eat.

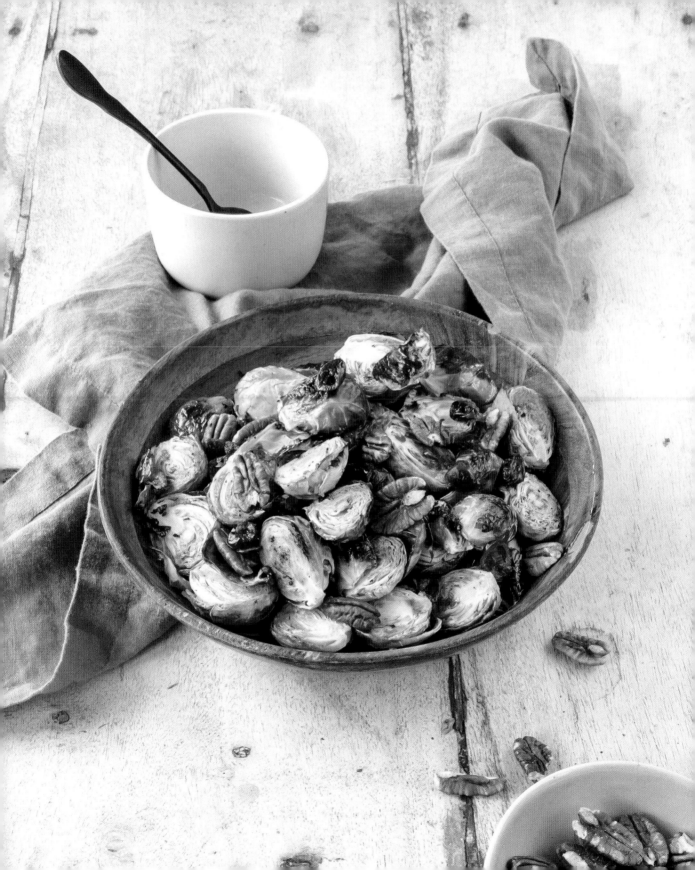

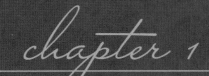

breakfast

Blueberry Breakfast Cookies | 37

Veggie Egg Cups | 38

Gluten-Free Protein Pancakes | 40

Maple Vanilla Overnight Oats | 42

HBE Breakfast Salad | 44

Cauliflower Hash | 46

Plant-Based Protein Waffles | 48

Hard-Boiled Egg Plate with Roasted Veggies | 50

Apple Blueberry Baked Oatmeal | 52

Breakfast Burritos | 54

Cranberry Almond Granola | 56

Bacon & Egg Casserole | 58

Maple Almond Baked Oatmeal | 60

Carrot Breakfast Cake | 62

Broccoli Potato Hash | 64

blueberry
breakfast cookies

2 medium overripe bananas

2 cups old-fashioned oats

½ cup almond butter

½ cup blueberries

¼ to ⅓ cup granulated sugar

1 scoop protein powder (optional)

1 teaspoon vanilla extract

½ teaspoon ground cinnamon

½ teaspoon coarse sea salt

meal prep tip:

Make these cookies in advance to have for breakfast or snacks throughout the week. They will keep in a sealed container in the refrigerator for up to a week.

I recommend using only ¼ cup of sugar to sweeten these cookies, but you can make them dessert cookies by using up to ⅓ cup of sugar if you like. You could also substitute powdered stevia or another sugar replacement in the ratio suggested on the label. (I find 3 tablespoons of stevia to be just right in this recipe.)

1. Preheat the oven to 350°F. Line a cookie sheet with parchment paper.

2. In a medium bowl, mash the bananas thoroughly. Add the remaining ingredients and mix well. Roll the mixture into 1-inch balls, place on the prepared cookie sheet, and flatten lightly with your fingertips.

3. Bake for 10 to 15 minutes, until browned. Enjoy warm right out of the oven or transfer to a cooling rack to cool before eating.

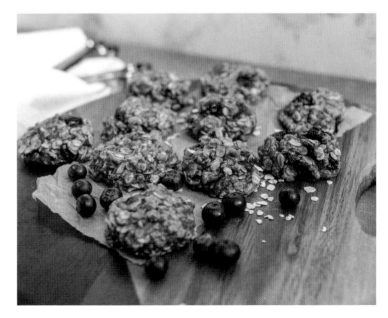

veggie egg

cups

YIELD: 8 egg cups (2 to 4 servings)
PREP TIME: 10 minutes
COOK TIME: 25 minutes

¼ cup finely chopped onions

1 tablespoon extra-virgin olive oil

1 tablespoon minced garlic

12 large eggs

1½ cups chopped fresh spinach

1 cup chopped red bell peppers

¼ teaspoon coarse sea salt

¼ teaspoon ground black pepper

¼ teaspoon ground dried thyme

1 cup crumbled goat cheese or other crumbled or shredded cheese of choice (optional)

SERVING SUGGESTIONS:

Salsa

Sliced avocado

The sautéed onions and garlic give these egg cups a savory flavor that you will love. You can add any veggies or cheese you like. You can even skip the cheese and make the egg cups dairy-free. They are especially good topped with some salsa and avocado slices.

1. Preheat the oven to 350°F and grease eight wells of a standard-size muffin tin.

2. In a medium skillet or sauté pan over medium-high heat, sauté the onions in the oil until they are translucent, about 5 minutes. Add the garlic and sauté for another minute, until fragrant. Transfer to a large mixing bowl and whisk in the eggs. Stir in the spinach, bell peppers, salt, black pepper, thyme, and cheese, if using.

3. Pour the egg mixture into the prepared wells of the muffin tin, filling them two-thirds full. Bake for 20 minutes, or until the tops are bubbling and the eggs are no longer runny. Serve hot topped with salsa and/or avocado slices.

meal prep tips:

Egg cups are easy to make ahead. They will keep in an airtight container in the refrigerator for about 3 days, so you may want to make a fresh batch midweek. I often make two batches since my husband and I tend to eat three or four egg cups at a time. Reheat them in the microwave on high for 30 seconds.

You can sauté the onions and garlic and chop the bell peppers up to 2 days prior to making the egg cups. Keep the prepared veggies refrigerated until you are ready to make the egg cups.

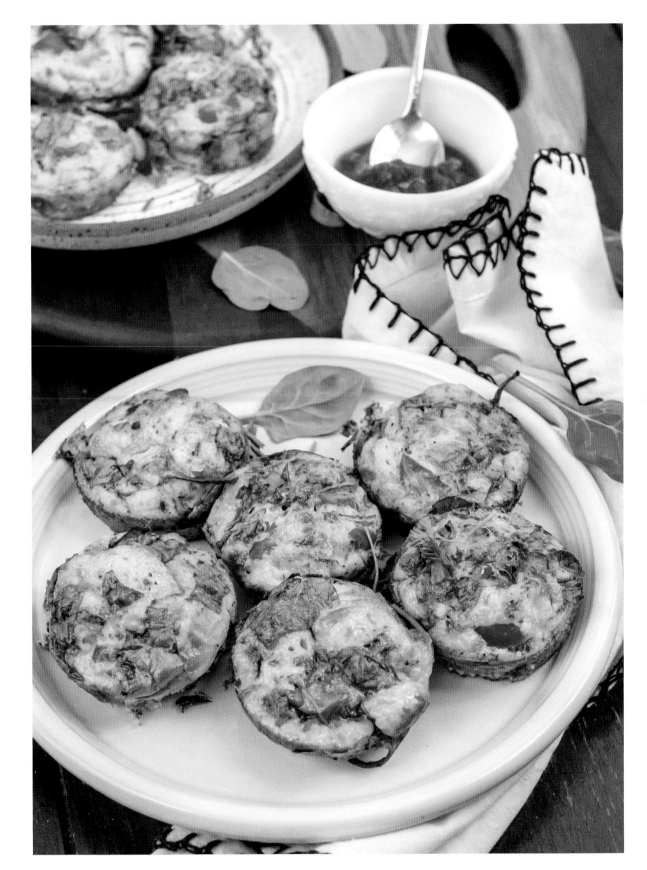

gluten-free
protein pancakes

YIELD: 16 (3-inch) pancakes (4 servings)
PREP TIME: 10 minutes
COOK TIME: 30 minutes

These are not your average empty-calorie pancakes. They are made with almond flour, and you can include protein powder so they offer more satiating calories throughout the morning than typical pancakes do. They are lightly sweetened, so you can go light on the syrup (or skip it entirely) and just top them with fresh fruit and some nuts or butter!

Because this recipe is made with almond flour, which can burn quickly, it requires close attention to detail. Follow the instructions closely for the best result.

2 large overripe bananas

6 large eggs

2 tablespoons maple syrup or honey

2 teaspoons vanilla extract

3 cups blanched almond flour

¼ cup protein powder (optional)

2 teaspoons baking powder

2 teaspoons ground cinnamon, for sprinkling

FOR TOPPING (OPTIONAL):

Fresh fruit

Maple syrup

Nuts and/or butter

1. Mash the bananas in a large mixing bowl. You should have about 1 cup of mashed banana, but a little more is fine. Whisk in the eggs, maple syrup, and vanilla, whisking well to eliminate most of the chunks.

2. In another large bowl, whisk together the almond flour, protein powder (if using), and baking powder. Get all the clumps out. Add the dry mixture to the wet ingredients and mix until thoroughly combined.

3. Heat a large skillet or griddle over medium-low heat. Grease the pan well.

4. Working in batches, scoop ¼ cup of the batter onto the hot pan. Use the back of a spoon to spread the batter into a 3-inch circle to ensure it cooks evenly. Repeat with two or three more scoops of batter.

5. Cook until the bottoms of the pancakes are golden brown and a few bubbles form on top, 2 to 3 minutes. Gently flip and cook until golden brown on the other side, 2 to 3 minutes longer (see tip). Remove the pancakes to a plate and repeat with the remaining batter, regreasing the skillet after each batch.

6. Serve immediately, sprinkled with the cinnamon and the toppings of your choice.

 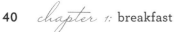

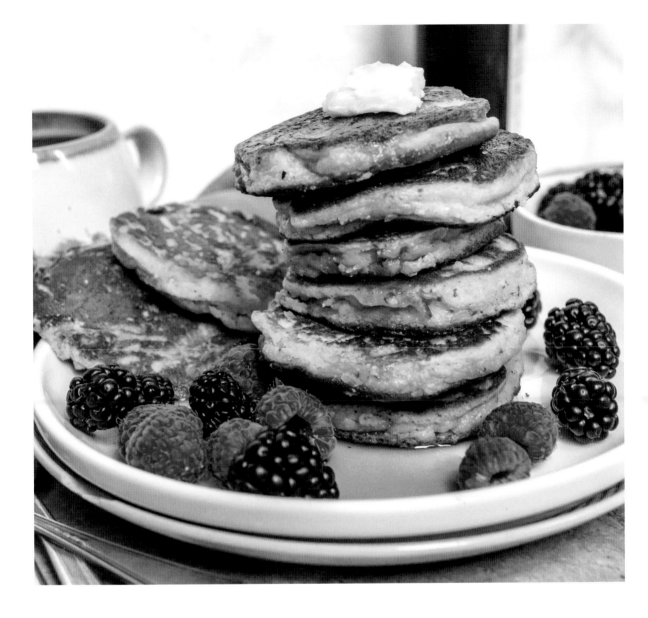

tip:

These pancakes can burn quickly, so be sure to check them frequently. If the pancakes start to burn, lower the heat. If they stick to the skillet, you need more oil. If they don't hold together as they cook, turn up the heat a little bit.

meal prep tip:

Let the pancakes cool completely before storing in a resealable plastic bag in the refrigerator for up to 5 days or in the freezer for up to 2 months. They reheat well in a toaster oven or microwave.

maple vanilla
overnight oats

YIELD: 5 large servings

PREP TIME: 5 minutes, plus at least 4 hours to soak

This recipe is great if you have a sweet tooth. You can play with the toppings so your oats never get boring: nuts, nut butters, fruits, and sweeteners will all change up the flavor if you don't like eating the same breakfast on repeat. I prefer my overnight oats at room temperature, so I take a serving out of the fridge about 15 minutes before I plan to eat it, but you can eat your oats cold or warm them up in the microwave if you like.

5 cups old-fashioned oats

½ cup plus 2 tablespoons chia seeds

5 cups So Delicious unsweetened coconut milk

3½ tablespoons maple syrup

5 teaspoons vanilla extract

Place the oats, chia seeds, coconut milk, maple syrup, and vanilla in a large glass or ceramic bowl and mix well. Cover and refrigerate overnight or for at least 4 hours before serving. Serve cold, allow to sit on the counter for 15 minutes to come to room temperature, or warm in the microwave for 30 to 60 seconds.

TOPPING OPTIONS:

Sliced banana

Blueberries

Chopped nuts, nut butter, or natural peanut butter

Hemp hearts

Maple syrup

Ground cinnamon

meal prep tip:

Overnight oats were the easiest thing I first started meal prepping. In my opinion, the longer the oats sit in the fridge, the better they taste. So be sure to make them over the weekend so you can enjoy them throughout your busy week! Instead of refrigerating the entire quantity in one large bowl, you can divide the oat mixture among 5 small lidded containers before refrigerating overnight for easy breakfasts on the go.

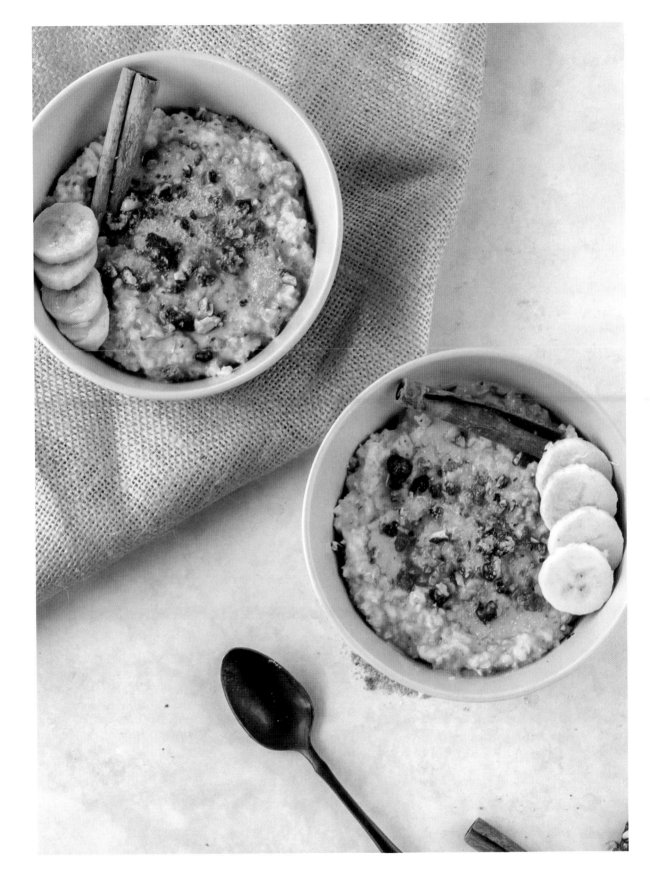

hbe breakfast
salad

YIELD: 5 servings
PREP TIME: 10 minutes (not including time to cook rice or quinoa)
COOK TIME: 20 minutes

2 medium sweet potatoes

10 large eggs

1 tablespoon white vinegar

2 teaspoons extra-virgin olive oil or avocado oil

½ cup chopped onions

1½ cups chopped broccoli

1 cup diced zucchini

½ teaspoon paprika

½ teaspoon garlic powder

½ teaspoon coarse sea salt

½ teaspoon ground black pepper

10 cups mixed greens, such as spinach, baby kale, or butter lettuce

1¼ cups cooked rice, such as RightRice, or quinoa

FOR GARNISH/SERVING:

Sliced avocado

Fresh herbs of choice

Salsa, hot sauce, or Cashew Queso (page 214)

I know it sounds weird to eat a salad in the morning, but trust me, this veggie-packed salad will leave you satisfied. The combination of eggs, avocado, and salsa or hot sauce makes it feel like you are at a diner, chowing on a healthy deconstructed burrito of sorts.

1. If desired, peel the sweet potatoes; if leaving the peels on, poke the potatoes several times with a fork. Microwave on high for 5 minutes. Remove and set aside until cool enough to handle, then dice the sweet potatoes.

2. Put the eggs in a large saucepan and pour in enough water to cover them. Stir in the vinegar. Place over high heat and cook for 10 to 12 minutes, including the time it takes for the water to come to a boil. Remove the eggs to a bowl full of ice water and allow to cool completely, then peel and slice them.

3. Meanwhile, heat the oil in a large skillet over medium heat. Add the onions and cook, stirring frequently, until softened, about 5 minutes. Add the sweet potatoes, broccoli, and zucchini to the skillet, then stir in the paprika, garlic powder, salt, and pepper. Cook, continuing to stir frequently, until the potatoes are nice and crispy on the outside, about 10 minutes.

4. To assemble the salad, put 2 cups of greens in a bowl, then layer with one-fifth of the veggie mixture, two sliced hard-boiled eggs, and ¼ cup of the rice or quinoa. Garnish with avocado slices and fresh herbs and drizzle with the sauce of your choice.

meal prep tip: ——————————————
To meal prep this salad, sauté the vegetables, hard-boil the eggs, and cook the rice or quinoa ahead of time, but wait to assemble the salad until you are ready to eat or leave for work.

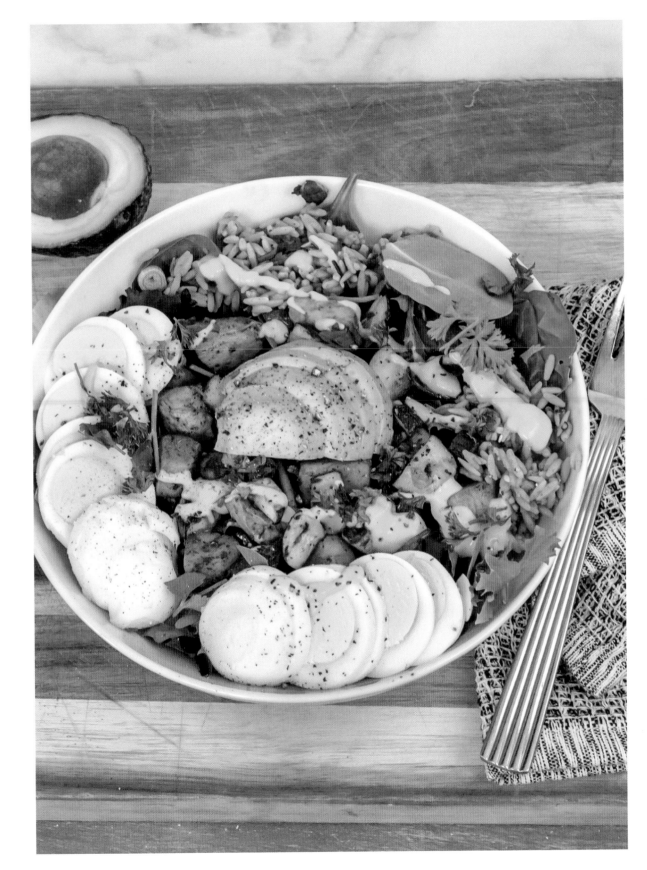

cauliflower
hash

YIELD: <u>4 to 6 servings</u>
PREP TIME: <u>15 minutes (not including time to fry eggs)</u>
COOK TIME: <u>15 minutes</u>

Cauliflower is having a moment! You can do just about anything with it. This hash is sure to become a new favorite of yours. You can serve it for breakfast or as a side to just about any main dish. I add a secret spice—which isn't so secret since it's listed here—to give the hash a unique flavor. Hint: it's cinnamon!

2 tablespoons extra-virgin olive oil

2½ cups chopped cauliflower

2 cups diced zucchini

½ cup diced onions

½ cup diced red bell peppers

1 tablespoon minced garlic

1½ teaspoons ground dried thyme

1 teaspoon ground dried oregano

1 teaspoon coarse sea salt

½ teaspoon dried marjoram leaves

½ teaspoon ground cinnamon

TOPPINGS:

4 to 6 fried eggs

Sliced green onions

Sliced or diced avocado

Salsa or hot sauce

1. Heat the oil in a large skillet over medium heat. Add the cauliflower, zucchini, onions, bell peppers, and garlic and sprinkle the thyme, oregano, salt, marjoram, and cinnamon over the veggies. Cook, stirring often, until the cauliflower is soft enough to be pierced with a fork, about 15 minutes.

2. Top each portion of hash with a fried egg, some green onions, avocado, and salsa or hot sauce and serve.

meal prep tip:

If you are meal prepping this hash for the week, add the fried egg to the hash the day you eat it, or pair the hash with hard-boiled eggs instead.

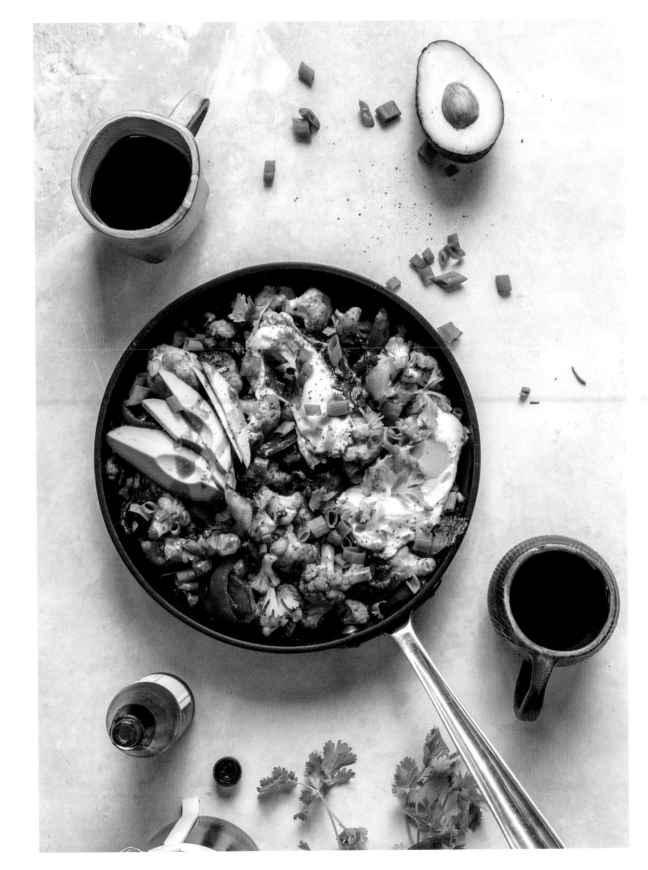

plant-based
protein waffles

YIELD: 4 Belgian waffles (4 servings)
PREP TIME: 5 minutes
COOK TIME: 20 minutes

These waffles are totally plant-based—no eggs needed! They are light and fluffy and full of flavor, but completely gluten-free so they won't weigh you down. If you don't have a waffle maker, you can make pancakes instead. I like to use stevia or monk fruit to sweeten the batter a bit; I use less maple syrup on top that way. I also top my waffles with fresh fruit to up the nutrients and antioxidants.

2 cups blanched almond flour, plus more if needed

¼ cup plus 2 tablespoons arrowroot starch or cornstarch

2 tablespoons baking powder

1 teaspoon ground cinnamon (optional)

½ teaspoon coarse sea salt

⅔ cup So Delicious unsweetened coconut milk, plus more if needed

3 tablespoons maple syrup, or 1 tablespoon monkfruit or powdered stevia

2 tablespoons extra-virgin olive oil

1 teaspoon vanilla extract

SERVING SUGGESTIONS:

Berries of choice

Maple syrup

Natural peanut butter

1. Preheat a Belgian waffle maker.

2. Put the almond flour in a large bowl and whisk out any clumps. Add the arrowroot, baking powder, cinnamon (if using), and salt and whisk well. Pour in the coconut milk, maple syrup, oil, and vanilla and use a rubber spatula to mix well. The batter should have the consistency of a traditional waffle batter. If it's too thin, stir in 1 tablespoon of almond flour at a time to thicken it. If it's too thick, stir in 1 tablespoon of coconut milk at a time to thin it.

3. Grease the hot waffle maker, then pour in ¼ cup plus 1 tablespoon of the batter and cook until golden brown, about 5 minutes. Repeat with the remaining batter to make a total of four waffles.

4. Top the waffles with berries, maple syrup, and/or peanut butter and enjoy!

meal prep tip:

If you are meal prepping these waffles, I recommend doubling the recipe. Store the waffles in a resealable plastic bag in the refrigerator for up to 5 days or freeze them for up to 3 months. Reheat them in an air fryer or toaster.

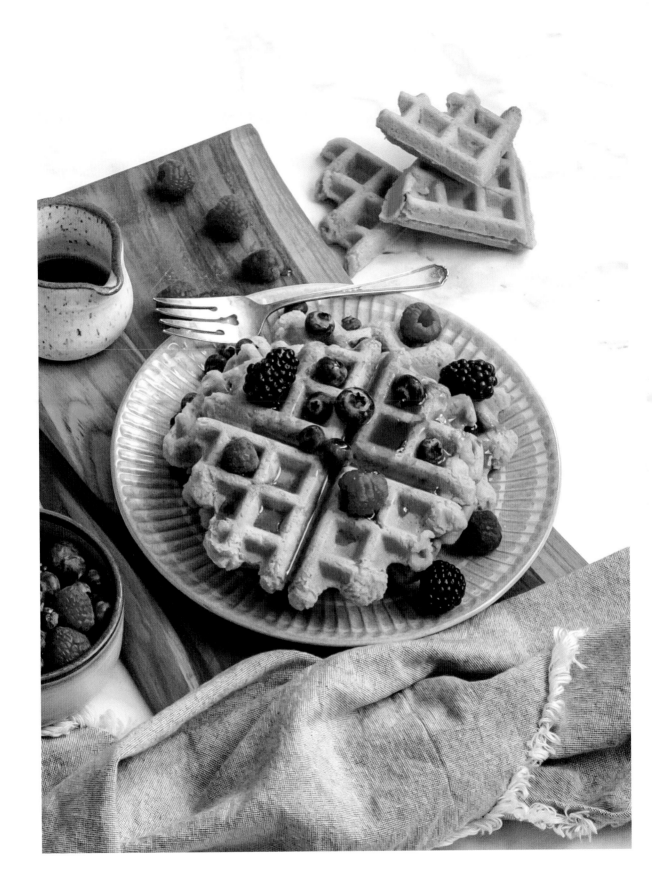

hard-boiled egg plate
with roasted veggies

YIELD: 4 servings
PREP TIME: 10 minutes
COOK TIME: 30 minutes

This is my go-to veggie-filled breakfast, and it's one of the MVPs on Sailorbailey.com. I love pairing eggs with roasted veggies, and I hope you do too. Breakfast is an opportune time to get those nutrients in! You can substitute just about any veggie you like if the ones listed aren't your favorites; this recipe is super customizable. When I want an extra hearty breakfast, I serve this with a side of cooked quinoa and some sliced avocado.

8 large eggs

1 tablespoon white vinegar

1 medium head cauliflower, chopped

3 medium sweet potatoes, peeled and chopped

1 medium red bell pepper, sliced

1 tablespoon minced garlic

1 tablespoon Italian seasoning

1 tablespoon paprika

½ teaspoon coarse sea salt

½ teaspoon ground black pepper

1 tablespoon extra-virgin olive oil

1. Put the eggs in a large saucepan and pour in enough water to cover them. Stir in the vinegar. Place over high heat and cook for 10 to 12 minutes, including the time it takes for the water to come to a boil. Remove the eggs to a bowl full of ice water and allow to cool completely, then peel them and slice them in half.

2. Meanwhile, preheat the oven to 375°F. Line a rimmed baking sheet with parchment paper.

3. Put the cauliflower, sweet potatoes, and bell pepper in a large bowl. Add the garlic, Italian seasoning, paprika, salt, and black pepper and toss well. Drizzle with the oil and toss again to be sure all the veggies are coated. Spread them on the prepared baking sheet and roast until tender, 20 to 25 minutes.

4. Serve each portion of roasted vegetables with two hard-boiled eggs.

meal prep tip:

For meal prep, divide the veggies among four containers and add two hard-boiled eggs per container. Store in the refrigerator for up to a week. If you have leftover veggies, you can toss them onto a bed of lettuce, drizzle with some dressing, and have yourself a delicious salad.

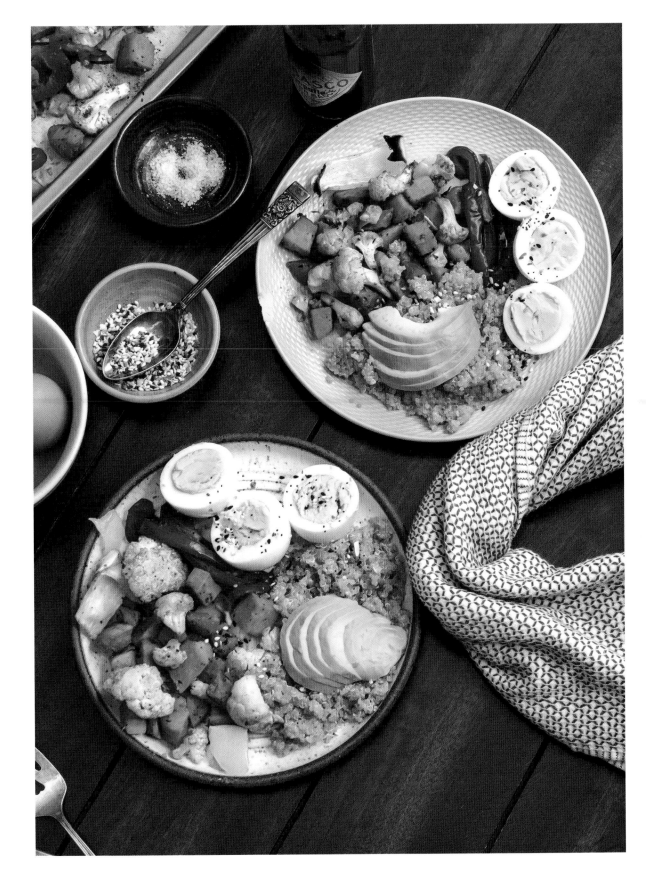

apple blueberry
baked oatmeal

YIELD: 6 servings
PREP TIME: 5 minutes
COOK TIME: 30 minutes

Cue all the cozy vibes for this dish! Baked oatmeal is the ultimate comfort breakfast, and it's so healthy. This recipe is practically foolproof, and using nondairy yogurt makes it totally plant-based.

1½ cups So Delicious unsweetened coconut milk

1 cup So Delicious unsweetened plain coconut yogurt

1½ tablespoons maple syrup or honey

1 teaspoon ground cinnamon

½ teaspoon ground nutmeg (optional)

⅛ teaspoon coarse sea salt

3 cups old-fashioned oats

2 cups diced apples (any type)

1 cup blueberries

1. Preheat the oven to 375°F. Line a 9-inch square or similar-sized baking dish with parchment paper.

2. In a large bowl, whisk together the coconut milk, yogurt, maple syrup, cinnamon, nutmeg (if using), and salt. Stir in the oats, apples, and blueberries; mix well, making sure everything is evenly distributed. Transfer the mixture to the prepared baking dish.

3. Bake until a toothpick inserted in the center comes out clean, 25 to 30 minutes. Let cool a little, if desired, then cut into squares and enjoy.

meal prep tip:

This is a perfect dish to prepare ahead for the week. It gets better and better as the week goes on and reheats easily.

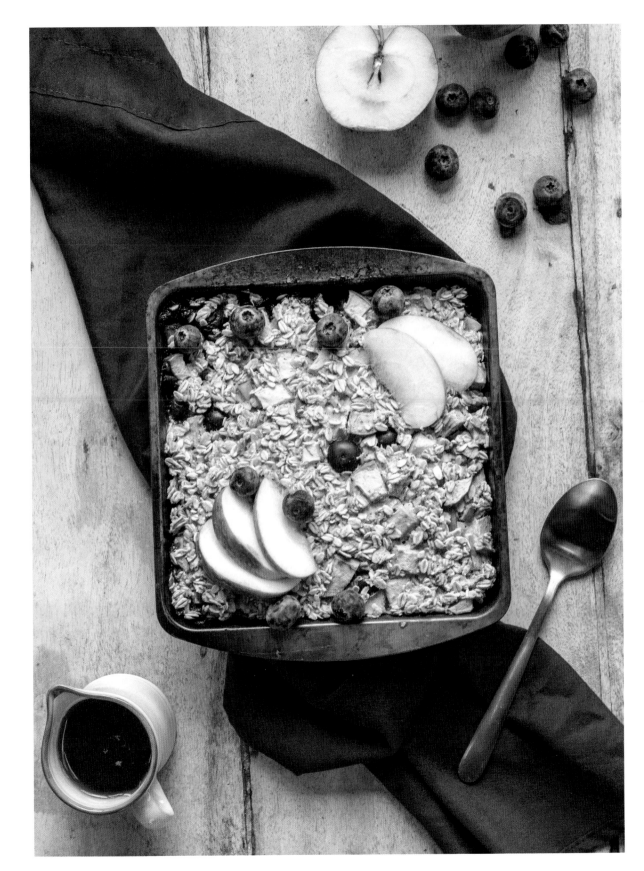

breakfast
burritos

YIELD: 4 to 8 servings
PREP TIME: 10 minutes
COOK TIME: 35 minutes

These burritos are full of veggies and protein from the eggs. You can add any cheese you like, but I usually go for goat cheese because it is easier to digest. Feel free to use up any leftover veggies you have in the fridge in addition to the ones listed here. For me, half a burrito is plenty, but those with larger appetites might want a whole burrito.

2 tablespoons extra-virgin olive oil, divided

1 cup diced russet potatoes

1 cup diced bell peppers (any color)

½ cup diced onions

½ cup finely chopped broccoli or cauliflower

½ teaspoon garlic powder

¼ teaspoon coarse sea salt

¼ teaspoon ground black pepper

1 cup canned pinto beans, drained and rinsed

4 large eggs

2 large egg whites

2 tablespoons water

4 burrito-size flour tortillas

3 cups chopped spinach

¼ cup shredded or crumbled cheese of choice

Sliced avocado, for serving

Salsa, for serving

1. Heat 1½ tablespoons of the oil in a large skillet over medium heat. Add the potatoes and cook, stirring often, until they start to soften up, about 10 minutes. Add the bell peppers, onions, broccoli, garlic powder, salt, and black pepper. Cook for another 10 minutes to soften the veggies, continuing to stir often, then mix in the pinto beans. Once the potatoes are fully cooked, transfer the bean and veggie mixture to a bowl and set aside. Wipe out the pan and set it back on the stovetop.

2. In another bowl, briskly whisk the eggs, egg whites, and water. Add the remaining ½ tablespoon of oil to the hot pan, pour in the eggs, and scramble over medium heat, about 3 minutes.

3. Layer the tortillas with the scrambled eggs, cooked bean and veggie mixture, spinach, and cheese. Do not overfill, or the burritos will not stay closed. Fold in the corners like a burrito and place back in the hot skillet. Brown the burritos on both sides, about 5 minutes per side, pressing them down with a spatula to keep them sealed as they cook.

4. Cut the burritos in half and serve with sliced avocado and salsa.

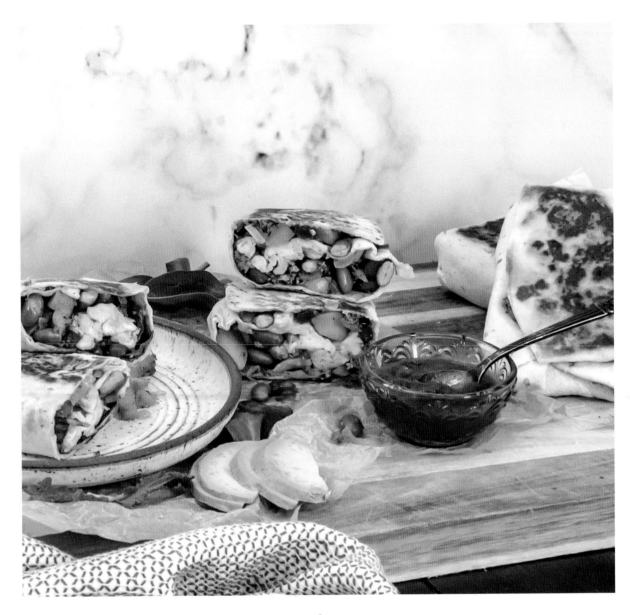

meal prep tip:

This recipe makes four large burritos that can be sliced in half and refrigerated for the coming week or frozen for later—the perfect meal prep breakfast for you and your partner! Wrap the burritos in parchment paper and refrigerate for up to 5 days or freeze for up to 3 months. If frozen, thaw in the refrigerator before reheating. When ready to eat, reheat the burrito in the microwave for 1½ to 2 minutes, until hot. You can cover it with a damp paper towel to keep the tortilla from drying out.

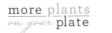

cranberry almond
granola

YIELD: 8 to 10 servings
PREP TIME: 10 minutes
COOK TIME: 45 minutes

You will never buy store-bought granola again once you realize how easy it is to make your own! You have more control over the amount of sugar, and you get to choose what goes into it.

3 cups old-fashioned oats

1 cup sliced or chopped almonds

½ cup chopped raw walnuts

½ teaspoon ground cinnamon

½ cup melted coconut oil

½ cup maple syrup or honey

½ teaspoon almond extract

1 cup dried cranberries

1. Preheat the oven to 300°F. Line a rimmed baking sheet with parchment paper.

2. In a large bowl, mix together the oats, almonds, walnuts, and cinnamon. In a separate bowl, stir together the coconut oil, maple syrup, and almond extract.

3. Pour the wet mixture into the dry mixture and stir well with a rubber spatula. Spread the mixture into a thick, even layer on the prepared baking sheet. Bake for 15 minutes, then gently turn the granola with a wooden spoon. Continue baking until the granola starts to brown and becomes fragrant, another 20 to 30 minutes.

4. Top the hot granola with the dried cranberries and let sit for 20 minutes to cool and harden before breaking it into chunks and serving or storing in an airtight container in the pantry for up to 2 weeks.

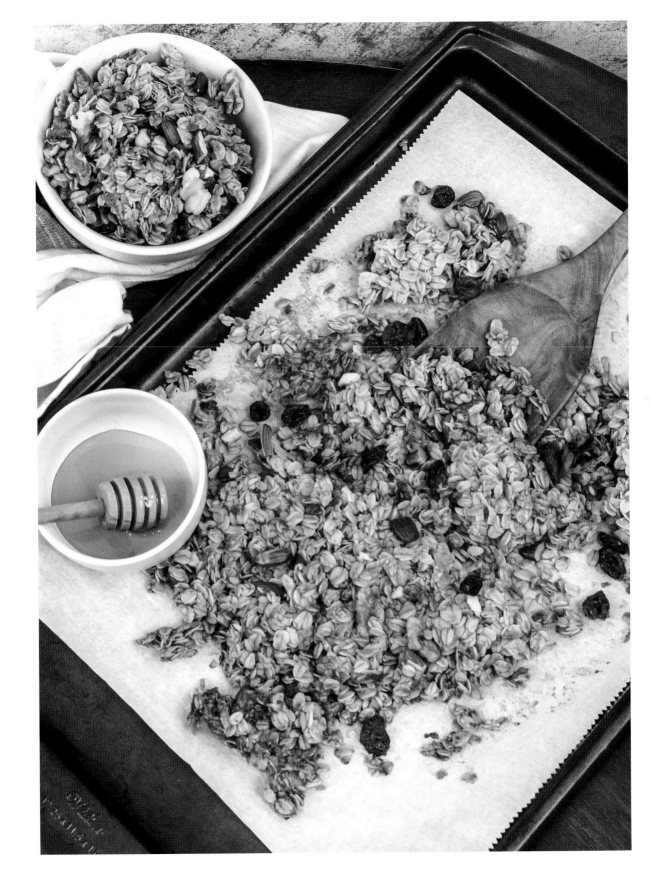

bacon & egg
casserole

YIELD: 6 servings
PREP TIME: 10 minutes
COOK TIME: 35 minutes

1 (16-ounce) package bacon

1 cup chopped zucchini

1 cup chopped bell peppers (any color)

½ cup chopped onions

1 cup chopped fresh spinach (optional)

½ teaspoon garlic powder

½ teaspoon coarse sea salt

½ teaspoon ground black pepper

10 large eggs

2 large egg whites

¼ cup water

This casserole is perfect for a meal prep breakfast or to feed a small army for a weekend brunch. It is packed with veggies, and bacon makes everything taste incredible!

1. Cook the bacon in a single layer in a large skillet over medium-high heat until browned and crispy, about 8 minutes. Remove the bacon to a paper towel–lined plate to drain. Keep 1 to 2 tablespoons of bacon grease in the skillet and discard the rest. You will be sautéing the veggies in the reserved grease.

2. Preheat the oven to 350°F. Lightly grease a 9 by 13-inch baking dish or similar-sized casserole dish.

3. Put the zucchini, bell peppers, and onions in the skillet with the bacon grease and sauté over medium-high heat until the onions are translucent, about 5 minutes. Add the spinach (if using), garlic powder, salt, and black pepper and sauté for 1 minute longer, until the spinach is wilted. Remove from the heat and let cool a bit.

4. Meanwhile, chop the bacon and set aside. In a large bowl, briskly whisk the eggs, egg whites, and water until frothy.

5. Add the chopped bacon and sautéed veggies to the bowl with the eggs and whisk well. Pour the mixture into the prepared baking dish and bake until the center is set, about 25 minutes. Let cool a bit, then cut into slices and serve.

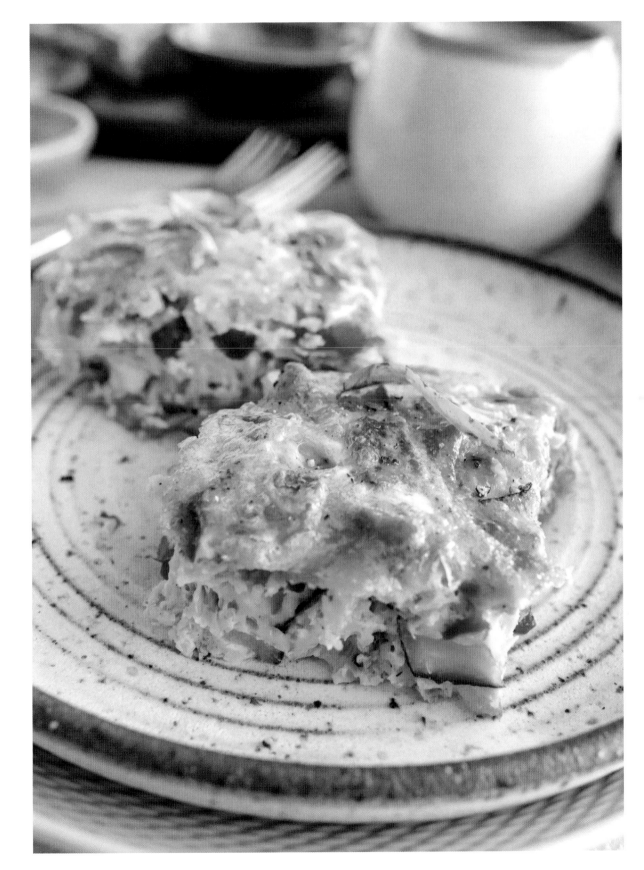

maple almond
baked oatmeal

YIELD: 8 servings
PREP TIME: 5 minutes
COOK TIME: 35 minutes

These nutty and sweet baked oats are easy to make and super satisfying. They also make a quick on-the-go snack.

2 small overripe bananas

1½ cups So Delicious unsweetened coconut milk

¼ cup almond butter

3 tablespoons maple syrup

1 teaspoon almond extract

1 tablespoon chia seeds or ground flax seeds

2½ cups old-fashioned oats

1 teaspoon baking powder

¼ teaspoon coarse sea salt

1 ripe banana, thinly sliced, for topping (optional)

¼ cup sliced or crushed almonds, for topping (optional)

1. Preheat the oven to 350°F. Grease a 9 by 5-inch loaf pan or line it with parchment paper.

2. Mash the bananas in a large mixing bowl. Stir in the coconut milk, almond butter, maple syrup, almond extract, and chia seeds.

3. Put the oats, baking powder, and salt in a separate bowl and whisk to combine. Add the dry ingredients to the wet ingredients and mix well.

4. Transfer the oat mixture to the prepared loaf pan. If desired, top it with the sliced banana and almonds. Bake until a toothpick inserted in the center comes out clean, about 35 minutes. Let cool a little, if desired, then cut into squares and enjoy.

meal prep tip:

The baked oats can be stored in an airtight container in the refrigerator for up to a week or frozen for up to a month. To reheat, wrap a square in a damp paper towel and microwave on medium heat for 30 to 45 seconds, or until warmed to your liking.

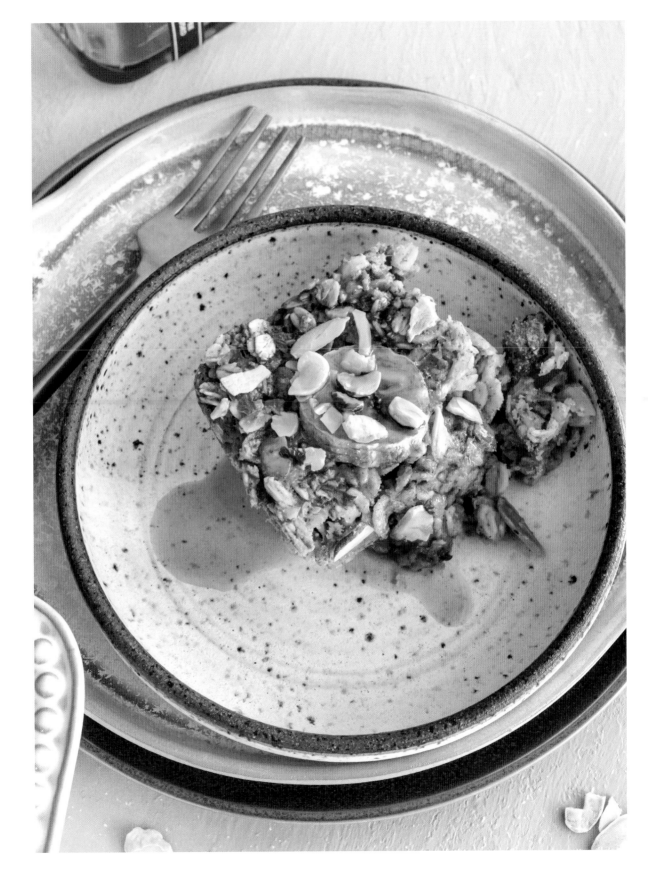

carrot
breakfast cake

YIELD: 6 to 8 servings
PREP TIME: 10 minutes
COOK TIME: 20 minutes

This cake is full of contrasting textures, warm spice notes, and carrots to boost your veggie intake. You won't feel guilty indulging in this light vegan cake—I need two servings on some days!

1 tablespoon chia seeds or ground flax seeds

2½ tablespoons water

2 cups old-fashioned oats

½ cup granulated sugar

1 tablespoon baking powder

1 tablespoon ground cinnamon, plus more for garnish if desired

⅛ teaspoon coarse sea salt

1 cup SILK unsweetened almond milk

½ medium overripe banana, mashed

⅓ cup shredded carrots

1 teaspoon vanilla extract

1 batch Vanilla Frosting (page 189) (optional)

1. Preheat the oven to 350°F. Grease a 9-inch square baking pan or line it with parchment paper.

2. Make the egg replacer: Combine the chia seeds and water in a small bowl; let sit until a gel forms, 5 to 8 minutes.

3. In a food processor, pulse the oats on high speed into a fine powder, about 3 minutes. Transfer the oat powder to a large bowl. Add the sugar, baking powder, cinnamon, and salt and whisk until combined.

4. In a separate bowl, stir together the egg replacer, almond milk, mashed banana, carrots, and vanilla. Add the wet mixture to the dry mixture and stir to combine.

5. Transfer the batter to the prepared pan and bake until a toothpick inserted in the center comes out clean, about 20 minutes. Let cool completely, then frost with the vanilla frosting, if desired. Cut into squares, garnish with cinnamon, if desired, and serve.

6. Store in the refrigerator for up to 5 days.

variation:

Pumpkin Spice Cake. Simply swap out the shredded carrots for an equal amount of pumpkin puree.

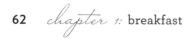

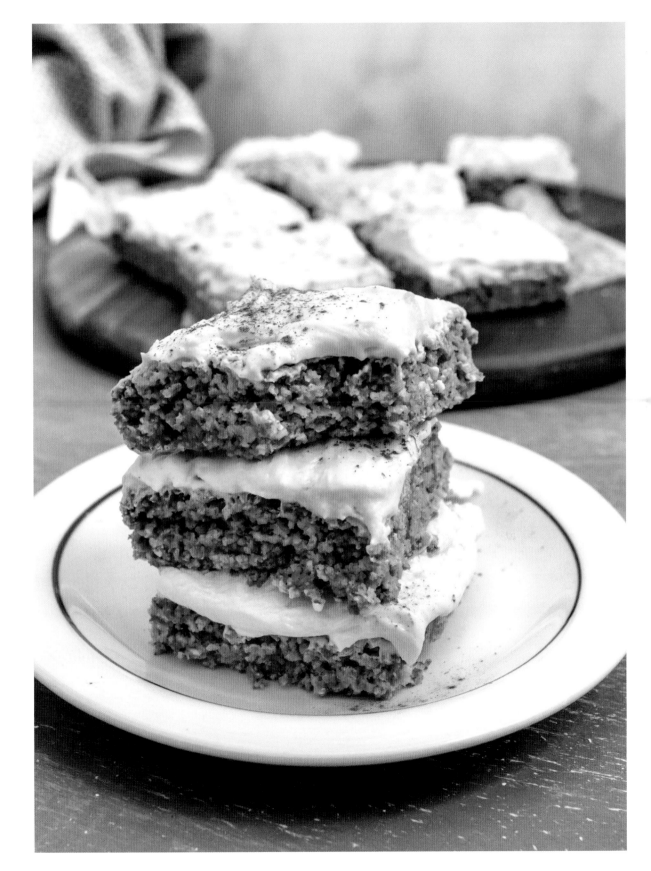

broccoli potato
hash

YIELD: <u>2 servings</u>
PREP TIME: <u>15 minutes</u>
COOK TIME: <u>20 minutes</u>

This flavorful hash is so easy to customize. For example, use a sweet potato or a russet potato, with or without the skin. Try zucchini instead of broccoli. Top the hash with a fried egg or a hard-boiled egg, or skip the egg altogether to make a vegan hash. If you want a sauce, I suggest hummus (see page 178; you may need to thin it with a bit of water) or one of the salad dressings in this book. Be sure to garnish your hash with tomatoes and avocado slices to boost your plant intake!

1 large sweet potato or russet potato

2 tablespoons extra-virgin olive oil or avocado oil, plus more for frying the eggs

½ cup chopped onions

2 cups chopped broccoli

2 cloves garlic, minced

½ teaspoon onion powder

½ teaspoon ground dried oregano

½ teaspoon coarse sea salt

½ teaspoon smoked paprika

¼ teaspoon ground cinnamon

2 large eggs

FOR GARNISH:

Halved cherry tomatoes or salsa

Diced avocado

1. Poke the potato several times with a fork. Microwave on high for 5 minutes. Remove and set aside until cool enough to handle, then peel and dice it.

2. Heat the oil in a large skillet or sauté pan over medium-high heat. Add the onions and sauté for 3 minutes. Add the diced potato, broccoli, garlic, and seasonings and stir well to thoroughly coat the potato and broccoli. Cook, stirring often, until the broccoli has softened and the potato is completely tender, about 8 minutes.

3. In a separate skillet over medium heat, fry the eggs in a bit of oil to the desired doneness. Serve the eggs on top of the hash and garnish with halved cherry tomatoes and diced avocado.

meal prep tip:

Prepare the hash in advance, heat it up, and top it with freshly fried eggs just before serving. You can also double the amount of hash and add the leftovers to salads or eat them as a side dish throughout the week. Leftover hash can be stored in an airtight container in the refrigerator for up to a week.

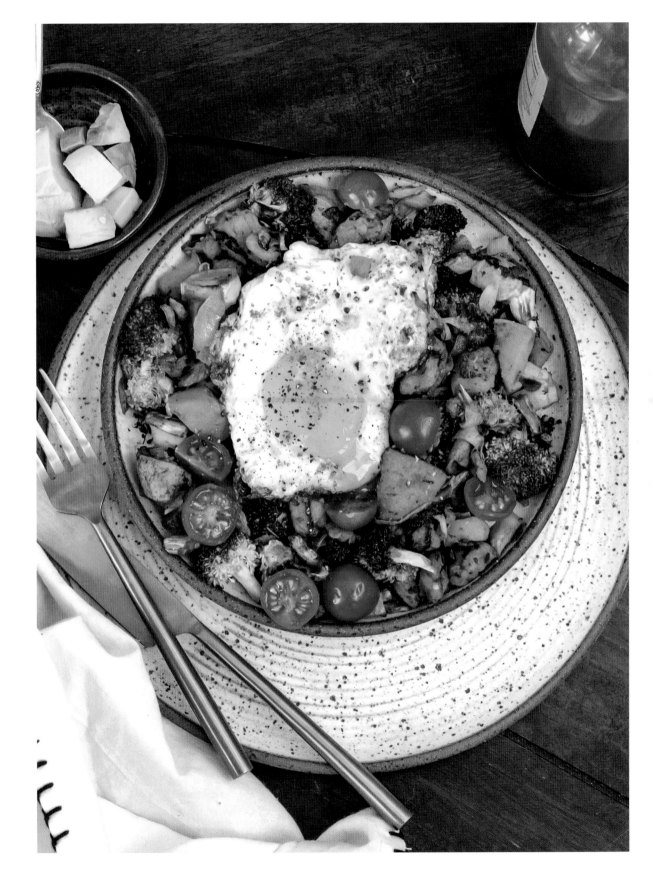

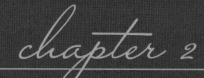

meatless mains

Veggie Taco Bowls | 67

Zucchini Parm Boats | 70

Zoodles with Artichoke Pesto & Mushrooms | 72

Broccoli Cheese Twice-Baked Potatoes | 74

Chipotle Acorn Squash & Kale Stew | 76

Cauliflower Curry | 78

Mushroom Stroganoff | 80

Loaded Black Bean Quesadillas | 82

Sweet Potato Burgers | 84

Plant-Based Creamy Broccoli Casserole | 86

Portobello Mushroom Burgers with Broccoli Slaw | 88

Creamy Fettuccine with Avocado | 90

Zucchini Lasagna with Plant-Based Ricotta | 92

Mushroom & Spinach Enchiladas with Cashew Queso | 94

Artichoke Zucchini Pasta with Roasted Red Pepper Sauce | 96

Baked Falafel-Style Balls | 98

veggie
taco bowls

YIELD: 6 servings
PREP TIME: 15 minutes (not including time to cook rice)
COOK TIME: 8 minutes

This recipe is easy to customize and will please anyone in the house. (Who doesn't love tacos?!) You can boost the protein by adding ground turkey, tofu, or tempeh, but honestly, you may not need it with all the satisfying veggies and toppings in this bowl.

TACO SEASONING:

1 tablespoon garlic powder

1 tablespoon onion powder

1½ teaspoons chili powder

1½ teaspoons chipotle powder

1½ teaspoons paprika

½ teaspoon ground cumin

½ teaspoon coarse sea salt

FILLING:

3 tablespoons extra-virgin olive oil

3 large zucchinis, diced

1 large onion, sliced

4 cloves garlic, minced

1 (1-pound) bag frozen corn kernels, thawed

2 (15.5-ounce) cans black beans, drained and rinsed

3 cups chopped fresh spinach

6 cups cooked rice

FOR TOPPING/GARNISH (OPTIONAL):

4 cups halved cherry tomatoes

5 cups shredded lettuce

1 cup plain Greek yogurt or sour cream, divided

2 avocados, sliced or diced

Fresh cilantro leaves

Lime wedges

Salsa

1. Make the taco seasoning: In a small bowl, stir together all the ingredients. Set aside.

2. Make the filling: Heat the oil in a sauté pan over medium-high heat. Add the zucchinis and onion and sauté until softened, 3 to 5 minutes. Add the garlic and taco seasoning and sauté for about 1 minute. Stir in the corn, beans, and spinach and cook just until the spinach begins to wilt. Remove from the heat and set aside.

3. Divide the rice among six bowls. Top with the zucchini and onion filling, then add the toppings/fillings of your choice.

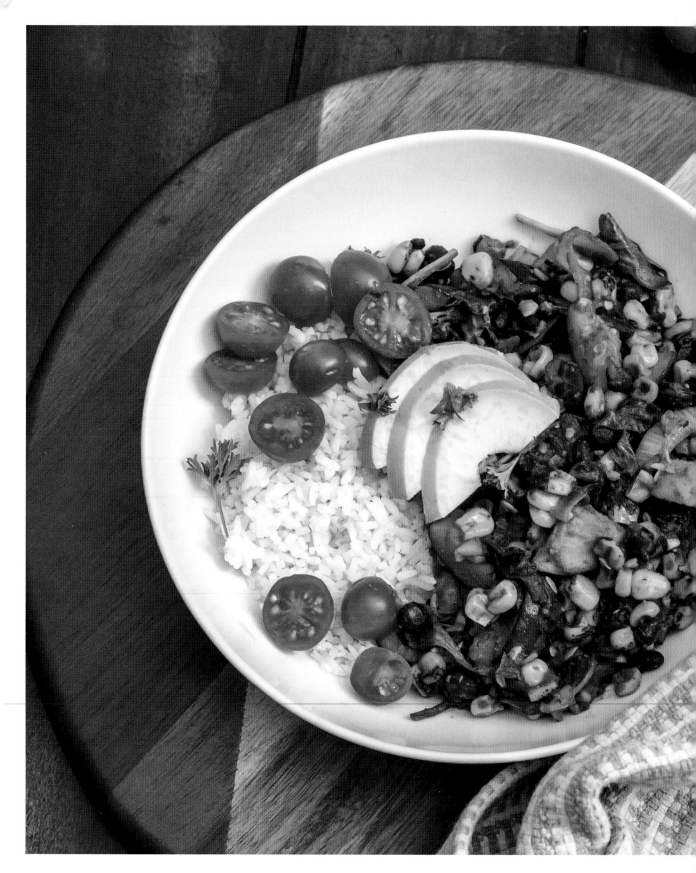

zucchini parm
boats

YIELD: 4 servings
PREP TIME: 10 minutes
COOK TIME: 25 minutes

Zucchini and summer squash are among my favorite vegetables to incorporate into meals. They are mild in flavor and texture and blend nicely with just about everything—even some sweeter baked goods. This recipe calls for zucchini, but you can use summer squash instead. My husband and I agree that this dish tastes similar to a much lighter version of eggplant Parmesan. You will love these boats for dinner, or as a cheesy side to any meal.

4 medium zucchinis

2 cloves garlic, minced

1 large egg

1 teaspoon Italian seasoning

½ teaspoon chili powder

½ teaspoon red pepper flakes

½ teaspoon coarse sea salt

½ teaspoon ground black pepper

½ cup plain breadcrumbs

¼ cup grated Parmesan cheese or Plant-Based Parmesan (page 212), plus more for garnish

¼ cup marinara sauce

½ cup shredded mozzarella cheese or vegan mozzarella

Thinly sliced fresh basil or parsley leaves, for garnish

1. Preheat the oven to 400°F. Line a rimmed baking sheet with parchment paper.

2. Cut the zucchinis in half lengthwise. Gently scoop out and discard the seeds. Scoop the fleshy center of each zucchini, making sure there is enough remaining flesh around the edge to hold the filling securely. Lay the fleshy parts on a clean dish towel, gather up the ends, and squeeze out all the liquid. Transfer to a food processor. Place the zucchini boats cut side up in the prepared baking dish.

3. Add the egg, Italian seasoning, chili powder, red pepper flakes, salt, and black pepper to the food processor and pulse to combine with the zucchini. Transfer to a bowl and mix in the breadcrumbs and Parmesan. Do not overmix; the stuffing should have some texture to it.

4. Spoon the stuffing evenly into the zucchini boats. Lightly spread the marinara over the stuffing, using about ½ tablespoon per boat. Sprinkle the mozzarella on top. Bake for 25 minutes, or until the cheese is bubbly and the zucchini is tender. Let cool for a bit before serving. Garnish with fresh basil and more Parmesan.

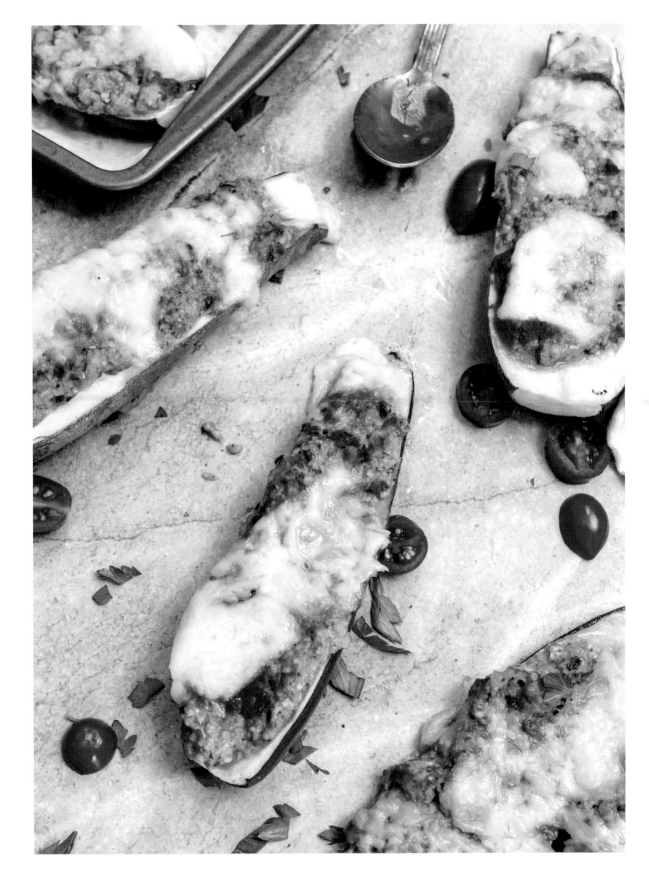

zoodles with artichoke
pesto & mushrooms

YIELD: 4 servings
PREP TIME: 10 minutes
COOK TIME: 10 minutes

If you haven't tried zoodles, please be open-minded; they are nothing like regular starchy noodles, but they are a great vehicle for a delicious sauce. They have half the calories of starchy noodles, so they leave you feeling lighter after a meal. You can use regular noodles in this recipe if you prefer. Feel free to adjust the basil, nuts, and/or salt to your liking as well. Pesto is very forgiving!

ARTICHOKE PESTO:

5 ounces fresh basil (about 2 big bunches), or ¼ cup dried basil, plus more for garnish

1 cup raw walnuts

¼ cup marinated artichoke hearts

¼ cup fresh spinach

¼ cup grated Parmesan or Pecorino Romano cheese, plus more for garnish

1 tablespoon chopped garlic

1 tablespoon fresh squeezed lemon juice

½ teaspoon coarse sea salt

¼ cup extra-virgin olive oil

1½ teaspoons extra-virgin olive oil

2 cups sliced mushrooms

4 cups zoodles (zucchini noodles)

Thinly sliced fresh basil leaves, for garnish

1. Make the pesto: Place the basil in a food processor. Add the walnuts, artichoke hearts, spinach, cheese, garlic, lemon juice, and salt and process until the ingredients are finely chopped but the pesto still has some texture to it; do not overblend. Scrape down the sides and blend again until there are no large pieces of nuts or basil.

2. With the motor running, add the oil in a slow, steady stream until the pesto is evenly blended. Scrape the pesto into a large mixing bowl; set aside.

3. Heat the remaining 1½ teaspoons of oil in a large skillet or sauté pan over medium-high heat. Add the mushrooms and cook, letting them brown without stirring too often, until they have a nice crisp to them, about 7 minutes. Remove the pan from the heat.

4. Add the zoodles to the bowl with the pesto; toss well to coat. Stir in the mushrooms and serve hot. Garnish with extra cheese and basil.

tip:

If you prefer your zoodles warm rather than raw, cook them in the pan in which you cooked the mushrooms over medium heat until warmed through, about 3 minutes.

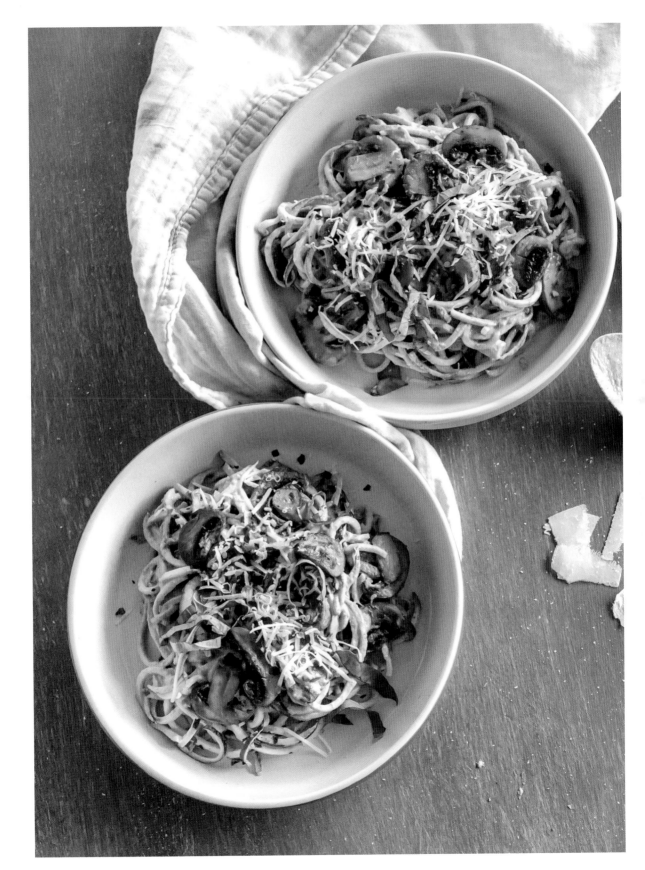

broccoli cheese
twice—baked potatoes

YIELD: 6 servings
PREP TIME: 30 minutes
COOK TIME: 1 hour 15 minutes

You can use either russet or sweet potatoes for this recipe. If you want more protein, you can add a pound of browned ground beef or turkey to the filling, but these potatoes taste just as good without meat. You can use vegan meat products if you prefer, and the results will be equally tasty.

6 medium russet or sweet potatoes

1 cup So Delicious unsweetened plain coconut yogurt or plain Greek yogurt

½ cup SILK unsweetened almond milk

3 tablespoons extra-virgin olive oil or unsalted butter

1 cup shredded or finely chopped broccoli

1 cup crumbled feta or goat cheese or shredded cheddar cheese, divided

8 green onions, sliced, green and white parts separated

1 clove garlic, minced

1 teaspoon ground dried oregano

½ teaspoon dried marjoram leaves

½ teaspoon coarse sea salt

½ teaspoon ground black pepper

1. Preheat the oven to 350°F.

2. Poke the potatoes several times with a fork. Bake directly on the oven rack until they are soft and can easily be pierced with a fork, about 1 hour. Remove from the oven and let cool for 10 minutes. Halve the potatoes lengthwise and scoop the flesh into a large mixing bowl. Arrange the skins on a rimmed baking sheet and set aside.

3. To the bowl with the potato flesh, add the yogurt, almond milk, oil, broccoli, ½ cup of the cheese, the white parts of the green onions, the garlic, oregano, marjoram, salt, and pepper. Mix with a hand mixer until creamy.

4. Spoon the broccoli-cheese mixture evenly into the reserved potato skins. Top with the remaining ½ cup of cheese and the green parts of the green onions. Bake until the cheese is browned and bubbling, about 15 minutes. Serve warm.

5. Store extras in the refrigerator for up to 5 days. To reheat, microwave for about 2 minutes.

meal prep tip:

I recommend prepping these potatoes on Sunday for the week. If you don't have time to make the whole recipe, bake the potatoes one night and then finish the recipe the next day.

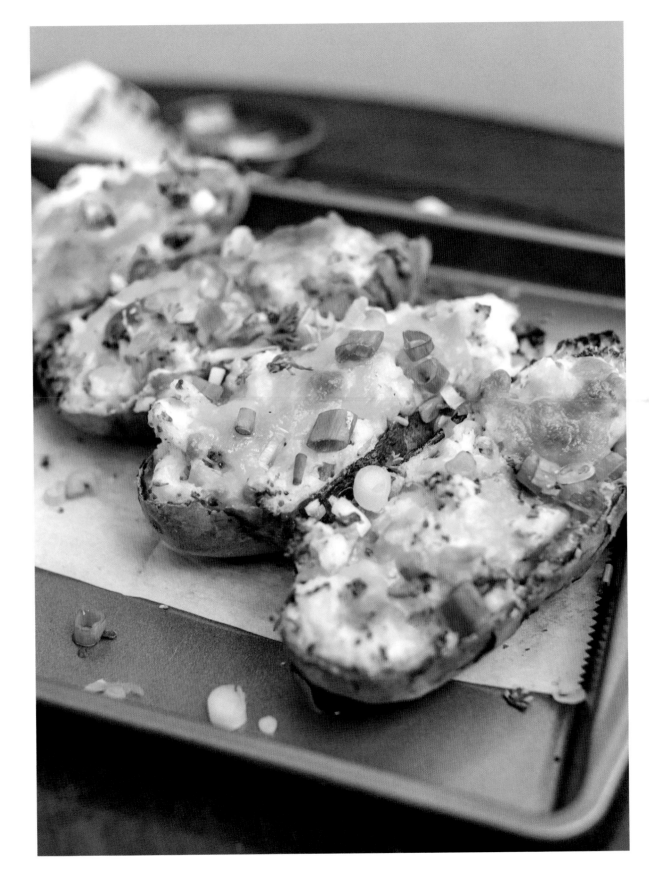

chipotle acorn squash &
kale stew

YIELD: 6 servings
PREP TIME: 15 minutes
COOK TIME: 4 hours

This stew has a sweet and savory vibe, and it is extra filling and cozy for cooler temperatures. You can easily add shredded chicken or ground turkey to increase the protein, but I prefer it as is with some shreds of nice Parmesan cheese on top. You can make this stew in a slow cooker to cook all afternoon or overnight, or you can cook it on the stovetop for an hour or two (but keep an eye on it, as the bottom can burn easily).

5 cups peeled and chopped acorn squash

5 cups stemmed and chopped kale

1 large onion, chopped

2 (15.5-ounce) cans light red kidney beans, drained and rinsed

1 (14.5-ounce) can diced tomatoes

1½ cups low-sodium chicken broth

1½ cups water

1 tablespoon minced garlic

1½ teaspoons coarse sea salt

1 teaspoon ground black pepper

1 teaspoon chipotle powder

1 teaspoon ground dried oregano

1 teaspoon smoked paprika

½ teaspoon garlic powder

Grated Parmesan or Pecorino Romano cheese, for garnish

Place all the ingredients in a 6-quart slow cooker and stir to combine. Cook on high for 4 hours or on low for 8 hours, or until the squash is soft enough to piece easily with a fork. Garnish with cheese and serve.

meal prep tip:

Prep this stew in advance and keep it in a large airtight container in the refrigerator all week. Garnish with the cheese just before serving.

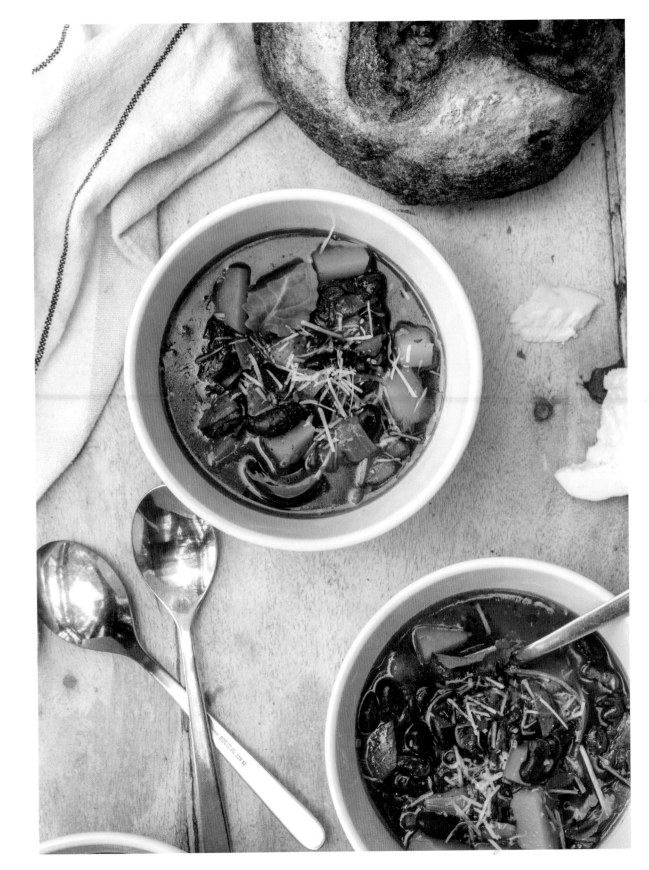

cauliflower

curry

YIELD: 4 to 6 servings
PREP TIME: 10 minutes (not including time to cook rice or noodles, if using)
COOK TIME: 25 minutes

This comforting dish is totally plant-based. The chunks of cauliflower and sweet potato give it a hearty texture, while the coconut milk gives it an authentic curry taste and highlights the other flavors in the dish. If you want protein, feel free to add some shredded chicken.

1 medium head cauliflower

2 tablespoons extra-virgin olive oil

1½ teaspoons curry powder

½ teaspoon garlic powder

⅛ teaspoon coarse sea salt

CURRY:

1 small sweet potato

1 medium red bell pepper, sliced

½ cup sliced onions

3 cloves garlic, minced

1 tablespoon grated fresh ginger

2 cups So Delicious unsweetened coconut milk, or more if needed to thin the sauce

½ (6-ounce) can tomato paste

2 teaspoons red curry paste

½ teaspoon cayenne pepper, or more if desired

½ teaspoon garam masala

½ teaspoon turmeric powder

1 teaspoon fresh squeezed lime juice

3 cups cooked rice or noodles, zoodles, or leafy greens, for serving (optional)

Fresh cilantro leaves, for garnish

Lime wedges, for serving

1. Preheat the oven to 400°F. Line a rimmed baking sheet with parchment paper.

2. Trim the cauliflower and chop it into florets. Place the florets in a large bowl and toss with the oil, curry powder, garlic powder, and salt. Spread the seasoned cauliflower on the prepared baking sheet and roast until tender and browned around the edges, about 15 minutes.

3. While the cauliflower is in the oven, make the curry. Poke the sweet potato several times with a fork. Microwave on high for 6 minutes. When the sweet potato is cool enough to handle, peel and dice it.

4. In a large saucepan, combine the diced sweet potato with the remaining curry ingredients and bring to a simmer over medium heat. Add the roasted cauliflower and simmer until everything is well blended, 8 to 10 minutes. If the sauce seems too thick, add a bit more coconut milk to thin it a bit. Remove the pan from the heat and stir in the lime juice.

5. Serve over rice, noodles, or leafy greens, if desired. Garnish with cilantro and serve with lime wedges.

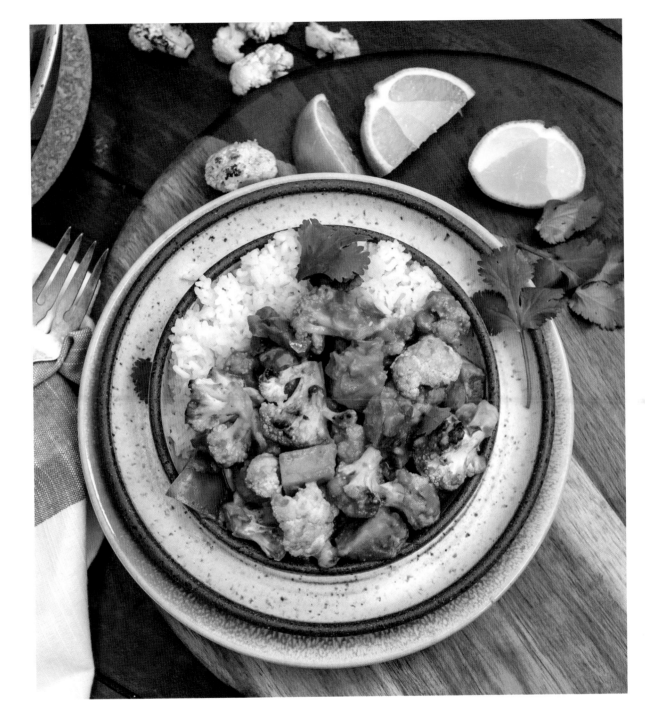

This dish is great warmed up throughout the week, so it's great for meal prep.

mushroom
stroganoff

YIELD: 4 to 6 servings

PREP TIME: 10 minutes (not including time to cook noodles)

COOK TIME: 15 minutes

This stroganoff is completely plant-based, and I can assure you that it is filling and extra tasty. Mushrooms offer such a good meaty texture; they are one of my favorite ingredients to bulk up any dish. You can serve this stroganoff over any type of noodle you like. I prefer eggless egg noodles, which are available at most major grocery stores.

2 tablespoons vegan butter

⅓ cup chopped onions

1 tablespoon minced garlic

1 tablespoon all-purpose flour (optional, for thickening)

5 cups sliced mushrooms (about 12 ounces)

2 cups low-sodium vegetable broth

¼ cup tomato paste

2 tablespoons vegan Worcestershire sauce or soy sauce

½ teaspoon dried thyme leaves

½ teaspoon coarse sea salt

½ teaspoon ground black pepper

¼ cup vegan sour cream

2 tablespoons SILK unsweetened almond milk

2 tablespoons chopped fresh parsley, divided

6 cups cooked noodles

1. Melt the butter in a large skillet or sauté pan over medium heat, then add the onions and garlic. Cook, stirring often, until the onions are translucent, 3 to 5 minutes. If you want a thicker sauce, whisk in the flour.

2. Add the mushrooms to the skillet. Cook for a few minutes, until they are tender, then pour in the broth. Bring to a simmer and stir in the tomato paste, Worcestershire sauce, thyme, salt, and pepper. Continue to simmer over low heat for about 5 minutes to allow the flavors to blend. Stir in the sour cream and milk and remove the pan from the heat. Stir in 1 tablespoon of the parsley.

3. Serve the mushroom stroganoff over the noodles. Garnish with the remaining tablespoon of parsley just before serving.

meal prep tip:

This dish will keep for about 5 days in the refrigerator and is great reheated. Just make sure to keep the stroganoff separate from the noodles.

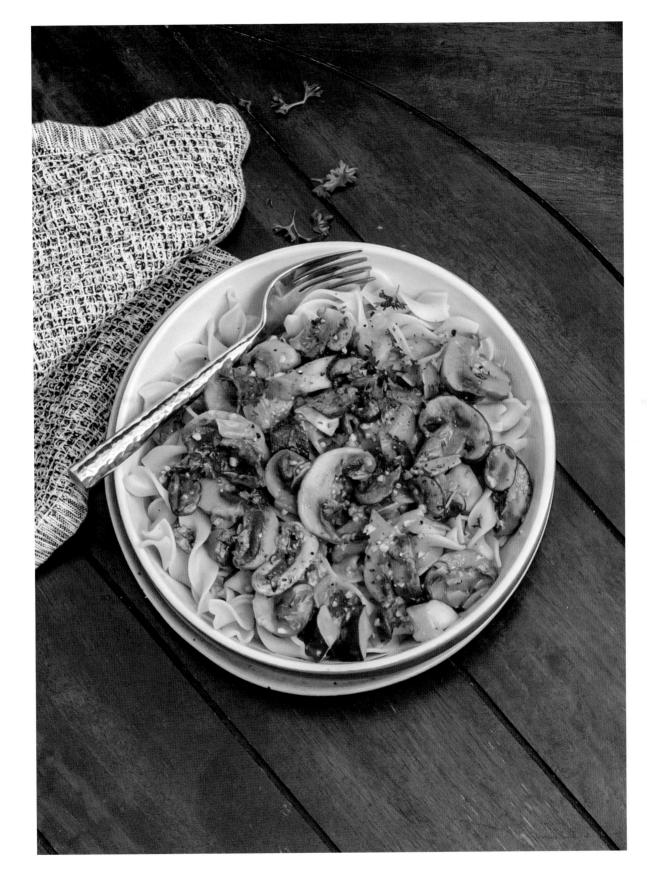

loaded black bean
quesadillas

YIELD: 4 servings
PREP TIME: 10 minutes
COOK TIME: 48 minutes

I've been making these quesadillas for some time, and they always hit the spot. They are not your average quesadillas! They're so packed with flavor, you would never guess they are completely plant-based. You can serve them for breakfast, lunch, or dinner, and my friends and family say that they are kid- and husband-approved.

1 large sweet potato

1 cup frozen corn kernels, thawed

½ cup canned black beans, drained and rinsed

¼ cup finely diced onions

½ (4-ounce) can diced green chilies (about ¼ cup)

2 cloves garlic, minced

½ teaspoon coarse sea salt

½ teaspoon chili powder

½ teaspoon paprika

¼ teaspoon ground cumin

4 (6-inch) flour tortillas

FOR SERVING:

Sliced or diced avocado

Sliced jalapeño pepper

Salsa

Vegan sour cream

1. Make the filling: Poke the sweet potato several times with a fork. Microwave for 6 minutes on high to soften it. Remove the skin, place the sweet potato flesh in a medium bowl, and mash with a potato masher. Add the corn, black beans, onions, chilies, garlic, salt, and spices; stir to combine.

2. Heat a skillet large enough to lay a tortilla flat in the pan over medium-high heat. Spray the skillet with cooking oil spray and lay a tortilla in the hot pan. Spread one-quarter of the filling mixture evenly over one half of the tortilla, fold the empty side of the tortilla over the filling, and press down lightly. Reduce the heat to medium-low and cook the quesadilla until crispy and browned on both sides, about 6 minutes per side. Repeat with the remaining tortillas and filling.

3. Top the quesadillas with avocado, jalapeño, salsa, and/or sour cream and serve.

tip:

If you prefer a heartier quesadilla, you can divide the filling among three tortillas rather than four.

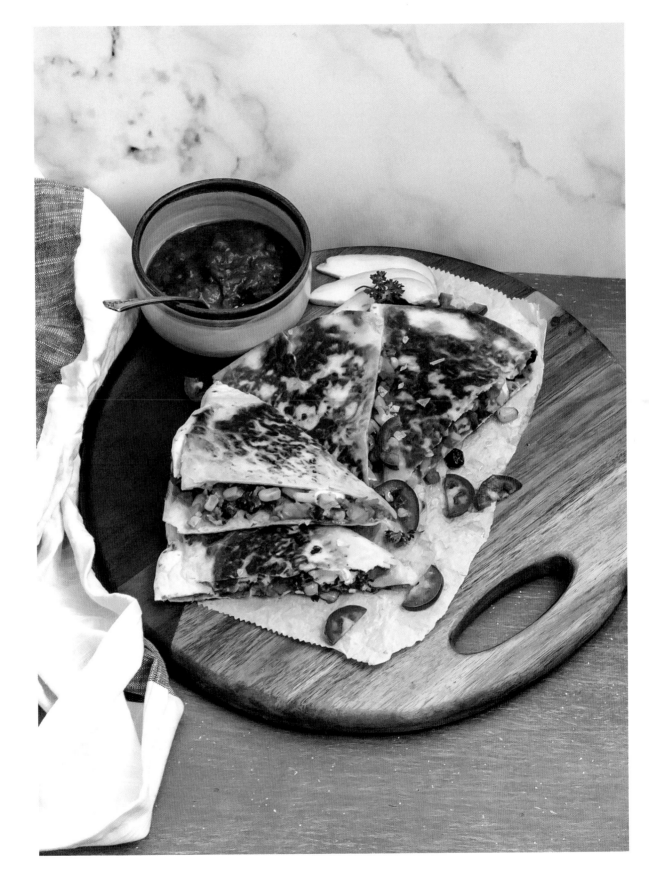

sweet potato
burgers

YIELD: 4 regular-size burgers or
6 slider-size burgers
PREP TIME: 15 minutes
COOK TIME: 45 minutes (not
including time to cook quinoa)

These flavorful burgers are fully plant-based and very
filling. They have a lightly sweet, smoky bite that will
leave you craving more! You can make them as sliders
or full-size burgers and serve them on lettuce leaves or
regular buns. These are thick patties; the thickness helps
them stick together better. Feel free to top your burgers
with cheese, onions, and tomatoes or however you would
dress a beef burger.

2 large sweet potatoes, peeled
and cubed

1½ cups cooked quinoa

1 cup canned black beans,
drained and rinsed

½ cup shredded carrots

½ cup panko or plain
breadcrumbs

½ cup finely diced onions

1 tablespoon chopped fresh
parsley

1 tablespoon brown sugar

½ teaspoon liquid smoke or
soy sauce

2 teaspoons smoked paprika

1 teaspoon garlic powder

1 teaspoon ground cumin

½ teaspoon chipotle powder

¼ teaspoon ground black
pepper

½ teaspoon coarse sea salt

FOR SERVING:

Butter lettuce or other sturdy
lettuce leaves, or regular or
slider-size burger buns

Burger toppings of choice

1. Preheat the oven to 400°F. Line a rimmed baking sheet
   with parchment paper.

2. While the oven is heating, put the sweet potatoes in a
   medium microwave-safe bowl, cover with plastic wrap,
   and microwave on high until soft, about 6 minutes. Add
   the quinoa, beans, and carrots and mash together, leaving
   some texture.

3. Add the panko, onions, parsley, brown sugar, liquid
   smoke, spices, and salt; mix well. Gently shape into
   1-inch-thick patties of the desired number and size
   (6 sliders, about 3 inches in diameter; or 4 full-size
   burgers, about 4 inches in diameter). Place the patties
   on the prepared baking sheet and bake for 25 minutes.
   Flip very gently and bake for another 15 minutes, or until
   browned and crispy on the outside.

4. Serve the burgers on lettuce leaves or buns, topped as
   desired.

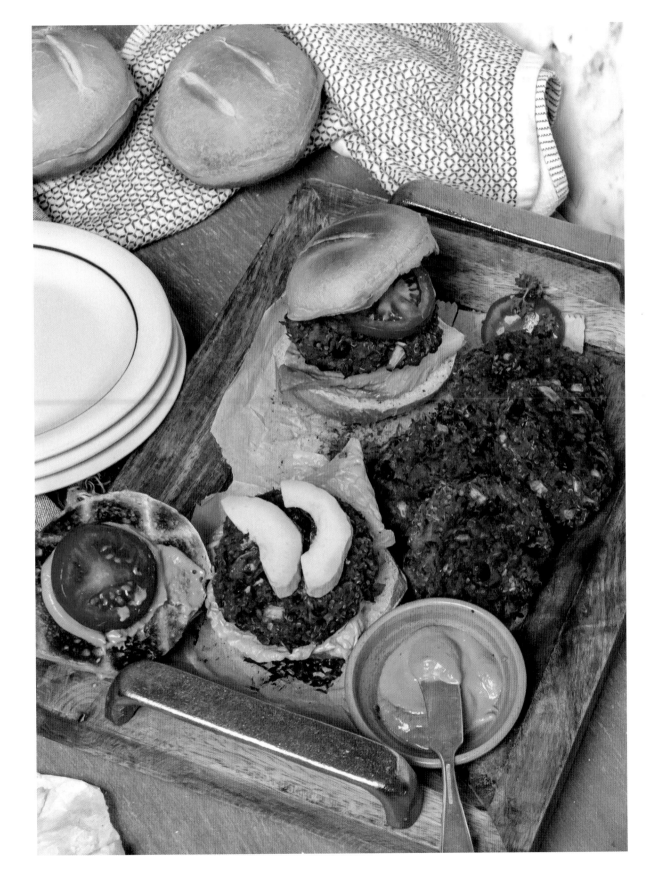

plant-based creamy
broccoli casserole

YIELD: 4 to 6 servings
PREP TIME: 10 minutes
COOK TIME: 43 minutes (not including time to cook rice)

This nourishing casserole is packed with flavor, and it only gets better throughout the week. You can use any kind of cheese, but plant-based cheese is a great option here; I find that Field Roast brand has the best melt. If you want more protein, add some rotisserie or grilled chicken.

6 cups chopped broccoli

1 cup sliced green cabbage

3 tablespoons vegan butter

1½ cups chopped onions

3 cloves garlic, minced

½ teaspoon chili powder

½ teaspoon ground dried oregano or Italian seasoning

½ teaspoon coarse sea salt

½ teaspoon ground black pepper

2 teaspoons arrowroot starch or cornstarch

1½ cups So Delicious Original coconut milk creamer

2 cups plant-based cheese shreds

TOPPING:

½ cup plain breadcrumbs or crushed crackers

½ cup plant-based cheese shreds

1 tablespoon melted vegan butter

1 teaspoon garlic powder

2 cups cooked RightRice or other rice of choice, for serving

Sliced avocado, for garnish

Chopped fresh parsley, for garnish

1. Preheat the oven to 350°F.

2. Bring an inch or two of water to a boil in a large saucepan over high heat. Insert a steamer basket, put the broccoli and cabbage in the basket, reduce the heat to a simmer, and steam the veggies until slightly softened, about 3 minutes. (You can also blanch them in a pot of boiling water for about 1 minute, then drain.) Transfer the broccoli and cabbage to a 9 by 11-inch or similar-sized casserole dish and set aside.

3. Make the sauce: Heat the butter in a large skillet or sauté pan over medium heat. Add the onions, garlic, chili powder, oregano, salt, and pepper and cook, stirring often, until the onions are translucent, about 3 minutes.

4. Lower the heat and stir in the arrowroot, making sure it is equally distributed. Pour in the creamer. Cook, stirring occasionally, until the sauce has thickened slightly, about 3 minutes. Add the cheese and allow it to melt.

5. Pour the sauce over the veggies, making sure the entire contents of the casserole dish are covered. Bake for 20 minutes.

6. While the casserole is in the oven, make the topping: In a medium bowl, combine all the topping ingredients. At the 20-minute mark, pull the casserole out of the oven and

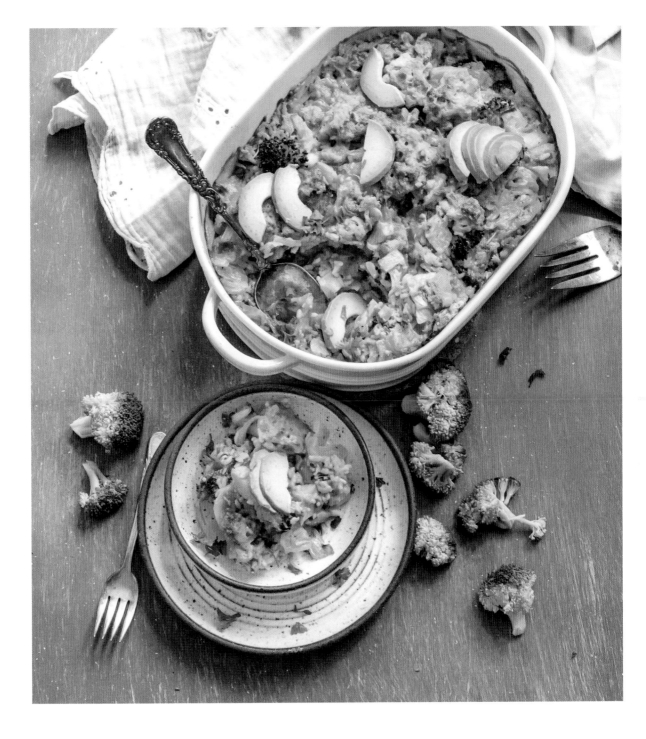

sprinkle the topping evenly over the casserole. Bake for 20 more minutes, or until the top is a beautiful golden-brown color. Serve with the rice and garnish with sliced avocado and parsley.

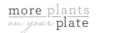

more plants
on your plate

portobello mushroom burgers
with broccoli slaw

YIELD: 4 to 6 servings
PREP TIME: 15 minutes, plus
15 minutes to marinate mushrooms
COOK TIME: 20 minutes

These mushroom burgers are so satisfying; you won't miss the meat. If you're not in the mood for slaw, you can pair these burgers with a side of my Sweet Potato Fries with Parmesan (page 162) instead.

4 to 6 portobello mushrooms, stems and gills removed

MARINADE:

¼ cup extra-virgin olive oil

¼ cup coconut aminos or soy sauce

1 tablespoon minced garlic

½ teaspoon maple syrup

½ teaspoon onion powder

½ teaspoon ground dried oregano

½ teaspoon dried thyme leaves

BROCCOLI SLAW:

1½ cups finely chopped broccoli crowns

1 cup coleslaw mix

¼ cup thinly sliced red onions

½ cup mayonnaise (regular or vegan)

2½ tablespoons granulated sugar

1½ tablespoons apple cider vinegar

½ teaspoon coarse sea salt

½ teaspoon ground black pepper

4 to 6 burger buns, or romaine lettuce leaves, for serving

1. Preheat the oven to 375°F. Line a rimmed baking sheet with parchment paper.

2. Put the mushroom caps in a large resealable plastic bag. In a small bowl, whisk together the marinade ingredients. Pour the marinade into the bag and let soak for 15 to 30 minutes.

3. Place the marinated mushroom caps on the prepared baking sheet with the stem side facing up. Pour the excess marinade into the caps. Bake until tender and darker in color, about 20 minutes, .

4. While the mushrooms are in the oven, prepare the slaw: In a large bowl, mix together the broccoli, coleslaw mix, and red onions. Put the remaining ingredients for the slaw in a separate bowl and emulsify with an immersion blender or whisk together well. Pour the dressing over the broccoli mixture and toss to combine.

5. Top the buns or lettuce leaves with the baked mushrooms and excess marinade. Fill the caps with broccoli slaw and enjoy!

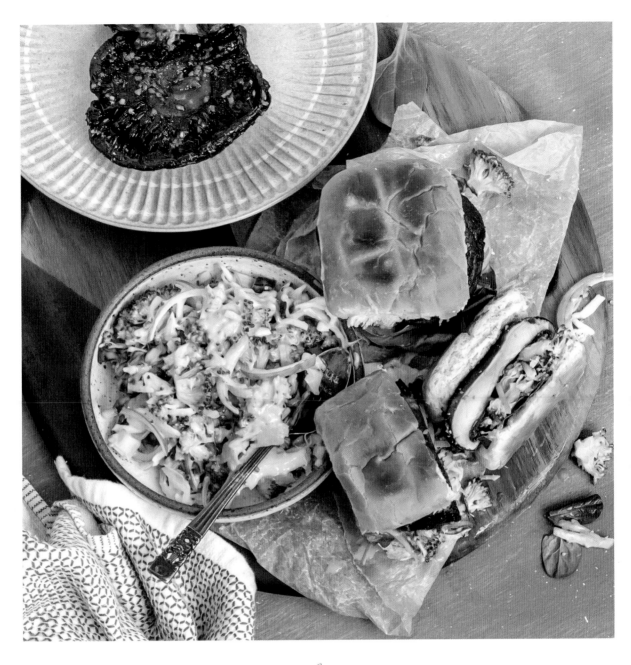

meal prep tip:

Make extra burgers for use in salads throughout the week; they are great sliced up on a hearty salad for a lighter meal. You may want to make extra broccoli slaw, too, to pair with these burgers, use as a side to one of my other fresh meals, or have on hand for a veggie-ful snack. It keeps nicely in the refrigerator for up to 4 days.

creamy fettuccine
with avocado

YIELD: 4 to 6 servings
PREP TIME: 10 minutes
COOK TIME: 15 minutes

This creamy vegetarian pasta calls for some fresh avocado slices on top. The avocado is totally optional, but it gives the dish a unique texture and flavor. You can make the recipe with zucchini noodles to up your intake of veggies here or use traditional pasta if you'd like more of a comfort meal.

1 pound fettuccine or other pasta of choice, or 3 large zucchinis, spiral-sliced into noodles

3 tablespoons unsalted butter or vegan butter

1½ tablespoons minced garlic

3 tablespoons arrowroot starch or cornstarch

1½ cups SILK unsweetened oat or almond milk

1 cup low-sodium vegetable broth

½ cup grated Parmesan or Pecorino Romano cheese or Plant-Based Parmesan (page 212), plus more for garnish

2 tablespoons fresh parsley, plus more for garnish

1 teaspoon fresh squeezed lemon juice

½ teaspoon coarse sea salt

½ teaspoon ground black pepper

½ avocado, sliced, for garnish

1. Cook the pasta in a pot of salted water according to the package directions. When done, drain and set aside. (If using zucchini noodles, you will add them to the sauce raw.)

2. Meanwhile, melt the butter in a medium saucepan over medium heat. Add the garlic and cook until browned, about 2 minutes. Slowly add the arrowroot, whisking briskly to prevent clumps from forming.

3. Whisking continuously, slowly pour in the milk and broth. Cook on a gentle simmer, whisking constantly, until the sauce thickens a little, about 5 minutes.

4. Add the Parmesan and whisk briskly until it melts completely. Stir in the parsley, lemon juice, salt, and pepper. Turn off the heat.

5. Add the pasta (or raw zucchini noodles) to the sauce and stir to coat. Serve garnished with avocado slices, more parsley, and more Parmesan.

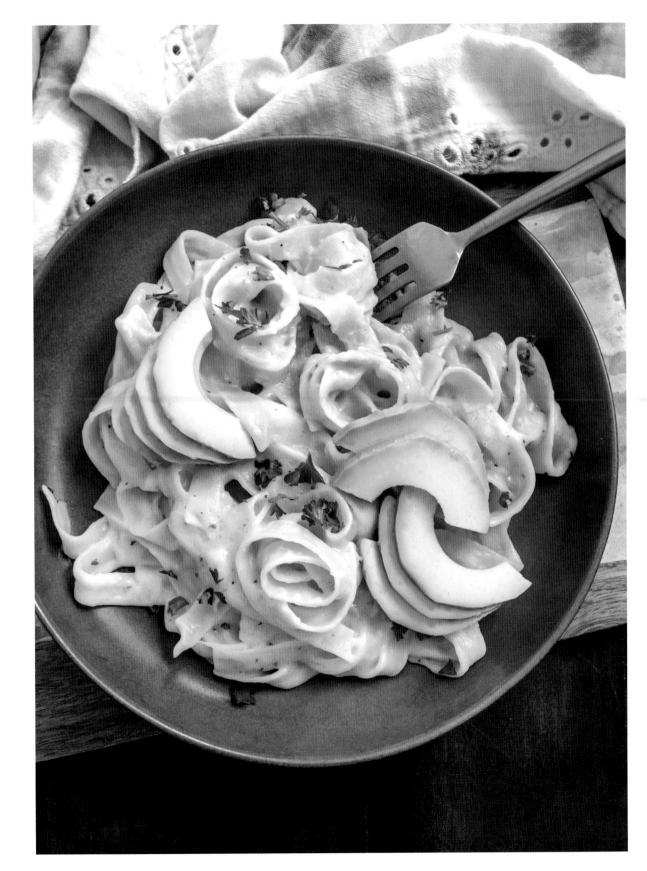

zucchini lasagna

with plant-based ricotta

YIELD: 4 to 6 servings
PREP TIME: 15 minutes
COOK TIME: 40 minutes

This veggie lasagna is not your average heavy comfort meal. It is filling, but it's a much lighter version of the Italian classic. As much as I love cheese, I like to cut out dairy where I can throughout the week, which is why I made this recipe totally plant-based. You can use dairy ricotta in place of the plant-based ricotta if you prefer. Use the full 3 cups of sauce if you like your lasagna saucy; otherwise, you might find that 2 cups is plenty.

PLANT-BASED RICOTTA:

1 (14-ounce) block firm tofu, drained

½ cup chopped onions

3 tablespoons fresh squeezed lemon juice

3 tablespoons nutritional yeast

2 cloves garlic, peeled

1 teaspoon ground dried oregano

½ teaspoon coarse sea salt

3 medium zucchinis (about 1 pound)

1½ teaspoons extra-virgin olive oil

¼ teaspoon coarse sea salt

¼ teaspoon ground black pepper

2 to 3 cups red pasta sauce, divided

1 cup sliced mushrooms, divided

1 teaspoon Italian seasoning, divided

1 cup vegan mozzarella shreds

¼ cup Plant-Based Parmesan (page 212), plus extra for garnish if desired

1. Make the ricotta: Put all the ingredients in a food processor or high-powered blender and blend to a smooth consistency similar to ricotta cheese.

2. Preheat the oven to 375°F. Line a rimmed baking sheet with parchment paper.

3. Slice off the ends of the zucchinis and discard. Cut the zucchinis lengthwise into thin, even planks (you can use a mandoline if you have one). Place the zucchini planks in a single layer on the prepared baking sheet. Drizzle with the oil and season with the salt and pepper. Bake for 10 minutes to soften them up.

4. Grease a 9 by 5-inch loaf pan or similar-sized baking dish. Spread 2 tablespoons of the red sauce on the bottom to prevent sticking. Layer the baked zucchini planks over the sauce in a single layer, then use a rubber spatula to smooth a thin layer of the ricotta over the zucchini. Add a thin layer of mushrooms and sprinkle with a pinch of Italian seasoning. Top with a drizzle of red sauce, then repeat the layers two more times, or until you have used all the ingredients. Top the last layer with the mozzarella and Parmesan.

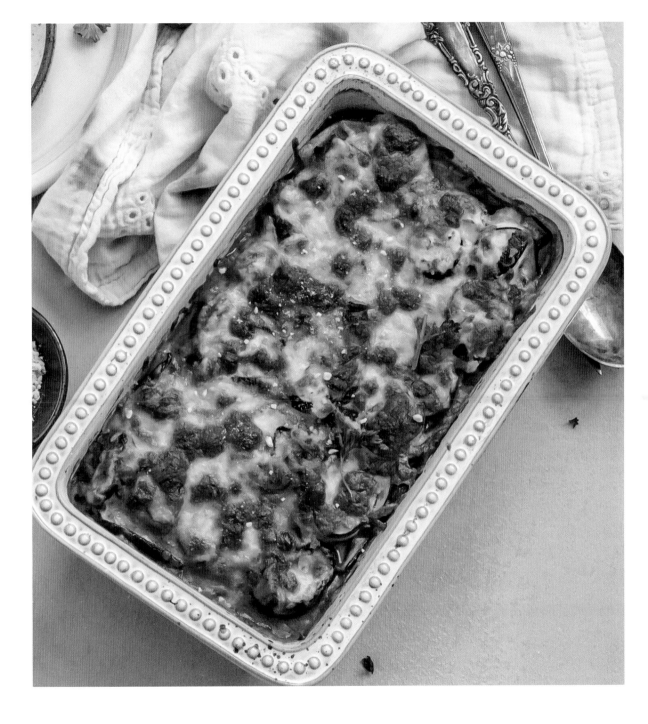

5. Bake until the sauce is bubbling and the top is golden brown, about 30 minutes. Let sit for a few minutes to cool and set before slicing and serving. Garnish with more Parmesan, if desired.

mushroom & spinach enchiladas
with cashew queso

YIELD: 4 servings
PREP TIME: 10 minutes (not including time to cook quinoa or rice or make queso)
COOK TIME: 28 minutes

This is a lightened-up version of the Mexican comfort dish. It has become my husband's favorite plant-based meal, which surprises me because he is a big meat eater! If you want additional protein, you can easily add some lean ground meat. However, if you think you need to add meat for flavor, trust me when I say it is not necessary. Move over, taco Tuesday; you have some enchilada competition!

1 tablespoon extra-virgin olive oil

3 cups chopped mushrooms

1 cup diced onions

1 cup cooked quinoa

1 tablespoon minced garlic

1 teaspoon chili powder

¼ teaspoon ground cumin

¼ teaspoon ground black pepper

⅛ teaspoon cayenne pepper

¼ teaspoon coarse sea salt

5 cups chopped fresh spinach

4 large or 8 small corn tortillas

1 (15-ounce) can enchilada sauce

Cashew Queso (page 214), for serving

2 cups cooked RightRice or other rice of choice, for serving

Sliced avocado, for garnish

1. Preheat the oven to 375°F. Grease a 9-inch square or similar-sized baking dish.

2. Heat the oil in a large skillet or sauté pan over medium heat. Add the mushrooms and onions and cook, stirring frequently, until the mushrooms are softened and the onions are translucent, 3 to 5 minutes. Add the quinoa, garlic, spices, and salt; stir to combine. Add the spinach and stir until it wilts. Remove the pan from the heat.

3. Divide the filling between the tortillas, roll each one up, and arrange, seam side down, in the prepared baking dish. Cover with the enchilada sauce. Bake until the sauce is bubbling, about 20 minutes.

4. Drizzle the queso over the enchiladas. Serve with the rice and garnish with sliced avocado.

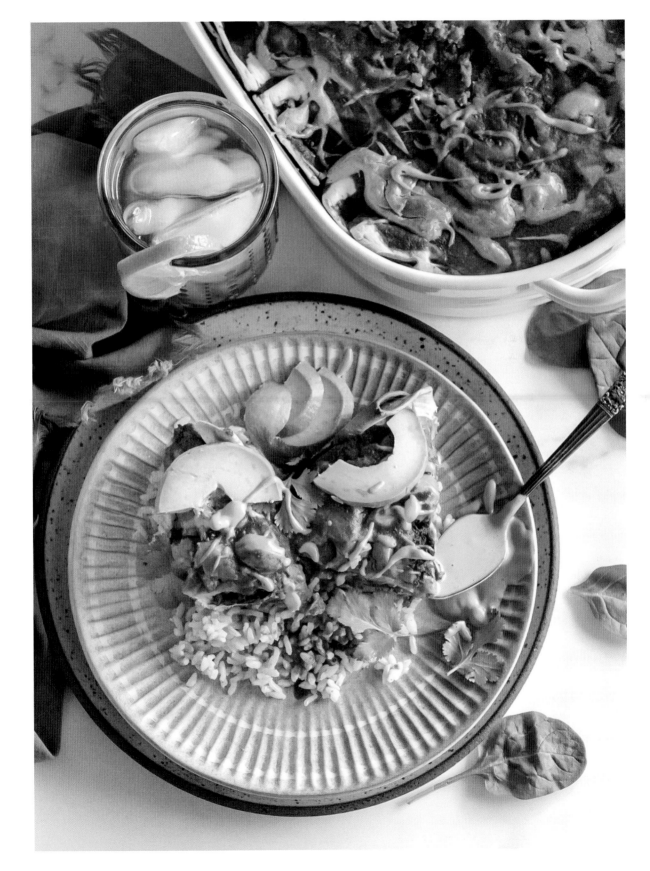

artichoke zucchini pasta
with roasted red pepper sauce

YIELD: <u>4 servings</u>
PREP TIME: <u>10 minutes</u>
COOK TIME: <u>35 minutes</u>

Mediterranean flavors meet Italian pasta in this savory and filling recipe. The roasted red peppers really bring this dish alive! You will love it on its own or topped with shrimp, chicken, or tofu for extra protein. It's also great paired with a salad and garlic bread. To save time, you can puree a 12-ounce jar of roasted peppers, drained, instead of roasting the peppers yourself.

2 red bell peppers

1 pound ziti or rigatoni

2 tablespoons extra-virgin olive oil

1 cup diced onions

1 cup chopped zucchini

1 cup marinated artichoke hearts, drained and chopped

4 cloves garlic, minced

½ cup tomato paste

¾ cup low-sodium vegetable broth

1 teaspoon coarse sea salt

2 cups chopped fresh spinach

½ cup So Delicious Original coconut milk creamer

Thinly sliced fresh basil leaves, for garnish

Grated Parmesan or Pecorino Romano cheese, for garnish (optional)

1. To roast the peppers, line a rimmed baking sheet with parchment paper, place the whole bell peppers on the prepared pan, and broil on high for 10 to 15 minutes, or until the peppers look charred and the skin is flaking off. Let cool, then remove and discard the skin, seeds, and stems.

2. Meanwhile, cook the pasta in a pot of salted water according to the package directions. When done, reserve 2 cups of the cooking water and then drain the pasta; set aside.

3. Heat the oil in a large skillet or sauté pan over medium-high heat. Add the onions, zucchini, and artichoke hearts and sauté until the veggies are sweating and fragrant, about 3 minutes. Add the garlic and sauté for another minute.

4. Add the tomato paste and cook, stirring often, for 10 minutes. (Tomato paste needs to cook up a bit so it isn't bitter.) The mixture will be thick. Add the broth and salt, bring to a boil, then reduce the heat to medium-low and simmer, stirring often, until the sauce has thickened slightly and the flavors are well combined, about 4 minutes.

5. Meanwhile, remove the stems and seeds from the roasted peppers and blend the peppers in a high-powered blender until smooth. Pour the peppers into

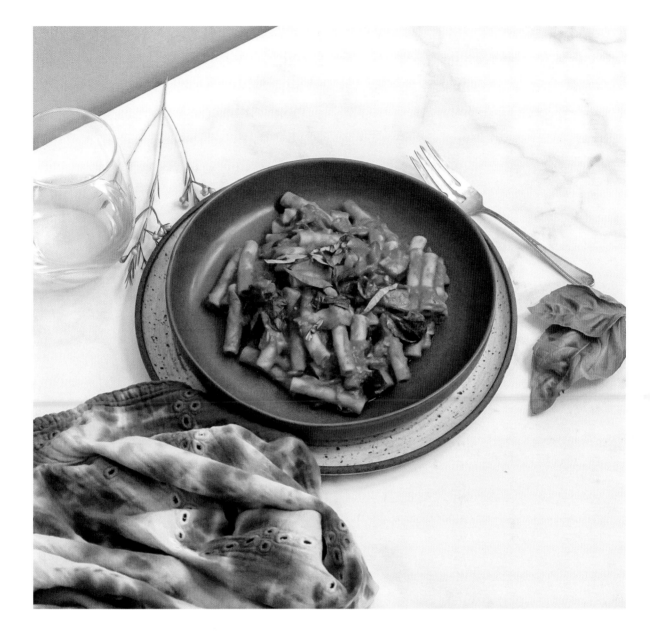

the skillet. Add the spinach, 1 cup of the reserved pasta water, and the creamer; mix well. Add more pasta water as needed to make the sauce pourable but still thick enough to stick to the noodles.

6. Add the pasta and toss with the sauce. Garnish with basil and cheese, if desired, and serve.

baked falafel-style
balls

YIELD: <u>4 servings</u>
PREP TIME: <u>10 minutes</u>
COOK TIME: <u>20 minutes</u>

These "meaty" vegetarian meatballs are full of texture and baked to crispy perfection. You can fry them, but I figure skipping oil where we can is always a plus. You can dress them up in your favorite sauce or enjoy them baked falafel–style with homemade hummus (page 178)—I have tried them both ways! I prefer them in the traditional Italian style, either on a sub or over pasta with red sauce, and my husband prefers them as falafel dipped in hummus. Choose your own adventure with these!

To make the prep work even faster, you can blitz the mushrooms, onions, garlic, and parsley together in a food processor.

1 cup finely chopped mushrooms

½ cup finely chopped onions

2 cloves garlic, minced

2 tablespoons finely chopped fresh parsley

1 cup cooked brown rice

½ cup old-fashioned oats

½ cup plain breadcrumbs

3 tablespoons Italian seasoning

1 teaspoon coarse sea salt

2 tablespoons soy sauce

2 tablespoons tomato paste

1 large egg, or 1 flax or chia egg (see page 10)

1. Preheat the oven to 375°F. Line a rimmed baking sheet with parchment paper.

2. Put the mushrooms, onions, garlic, and parsley in a large bowl. Add the cooked rice, oats, breadcrumbs, Italian seasoning, and salt and stir to combine. Add the soy sauce, tomato paste, and egg and stir well.

3. Use a small cookie scoop to form the mixture into ten 1-inch balls and place on the prepared baking sheet. If the mixture is too sticky, coat the scoop with olive oil to help prevent sticking. You can also add more breadcrumbs 1 tablespoon at a time if the mixture isn't holding together.

4. Bake the meatballs until golden brown and crispy on the outside, about 20 minutes.

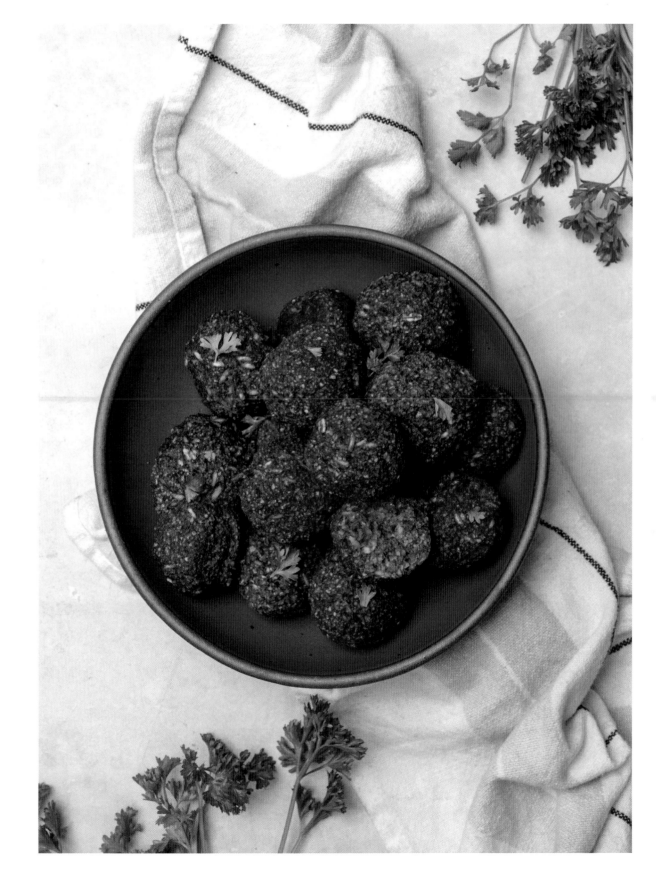

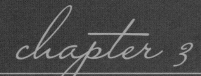

beef, chicken & turkey recipes

Garlic Dijon Chicken | 101

Turkey Veggie Meatballs | 104

Baked Ziti | 106

Chicken Tacos | 108

Sneaky Turkey Meatloaf | 110

Stuffed Peppers | 112

Three-Bean Turkey Chili | 114

Turkey Feta Meatballs with
Red Pepper Sauce | 116

Chicken & Veggie Sheet Pan Meal | 118

Shredded BBQ Chicken & Peppers | 120

Almond Cashew Coconut Chicken Tenders with Honey Mustard | 122

Chicken Sausage Fajitas | 124

Pepperoni Rigatoni | 126

Beef Spaghetti Squash with Tzatziki | 128

Turkey Veggie Tacos | 130

garlic dijon
chicken

YIELD: 4 to 6 servings

PREP TIME: 15 minutes (not including time to cook rice or noodles)

COOK TIME: 30 minutes

This dish is a crowd-pleaser! I've been making it for years, and my friends and family are always blown away by it. The Dijon mustard blends so nicely with the yogurt. For a less formal presentation, I sometimes like to cube the cooked chicken. It stretches the meal further and makes the chicken even tastier.

2 teaspoons seasoning salt

1 teaspoon garlic powder

½ teaspoon onion powder

1 teaspoon ground black pepper, divided

1½ pounds boneless, skinless chicken breasts or thighs

3 tablespoons extra-virgin olive oil, divided

4 cups chopped broccoli

2 onions, sliced

8 cloves garlic, minced

2 tablespoons chopped fresh parsley, plus more for garnish (optional)

2 teaspoons dried thyme leaves

2 teaspoons dried rosemary leaves

2 cups low-sodium chicken broth

1⅓ cups plain Greek yogurt or sour cream

1½ teaspoons Dijon mustard

1 cup chopped tomatoes, or ½ (8.5-ounce) jar sun-dried tomatoes in oil

1 teaspoon coarse sea salt

½ teaspoon red pepper flakes (optional)

4 cups chopped fresh spinach

4 to 6 cups cooked rice or noodles, for serving

1. In a large bowl, stir together the seasoning salt, garlic powder, onion powder, and ½ teaspoon of the black pepper until well blended. Add the chicken to the bowl and rub it with the seasoning mix until thoroughly coated.

2. Heat 1 tablespoon of the oil in a large skillet or sauté pan over medium-high heat. Add the seasoned chicken and cook until golden brown on the outside and cooked through, about 8 minutes per side, depending on thickness. Do not overcook. Transfer the chicken to a plate and set aside, keeping the skillet on the burner.

3. Add the remaining 2 tablespoons of oil along with the broccoli and onions to the skillet and sauté until the onions start to turn translucent, about 5 minutes. Add the garlic and herbs and cook for 1 to 2 minutes, until wilted and fragrant. Pour in the broth and use a wooden spoon to scrape up any bits from the bottom of the pan; simmer for 3 to 4 minutes, until the sauce is well combined and thickened.

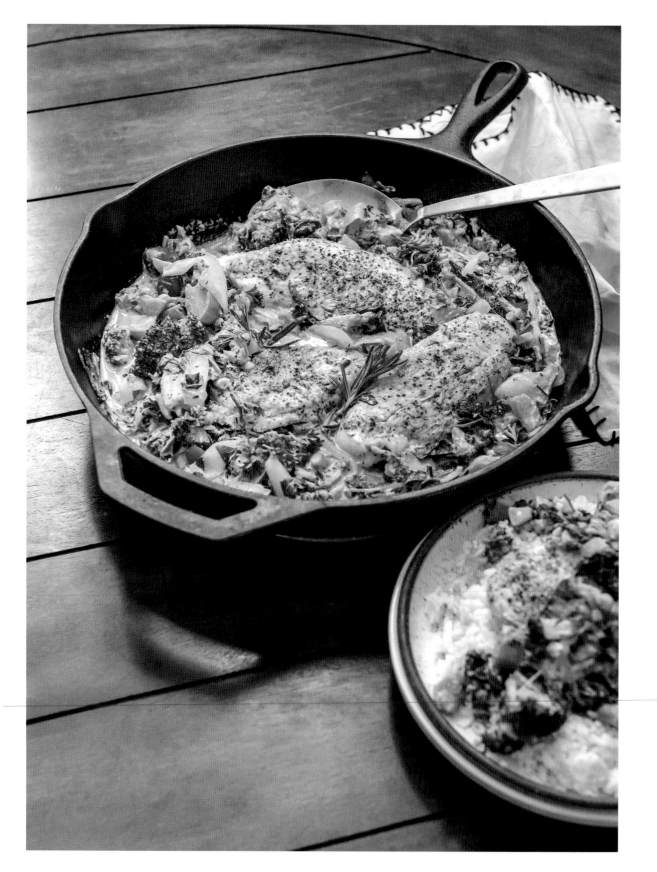

*To make this dish vegan, substitute 2 (14- to 16-ounce) packages of firm or extra-firm tofu for the chicken, substitute vegetable broth for the chicken broth, and use vegan sour cream. Cut the tofu into bite-sized pieces and cook it for about 6 minutes.

4. In a small bowl, whisk together the yogurt and mustard, then pour the mixture into the skillet. Bring to a low boil, then reduce the heat to a gentle simmer until the sauce thickens, about 2 minutes. Add tomatoes, salt, the remaining ½ teaspoon of black pepper, and the red pepper flakes, if using; stir, then mix in the spinach. If desired, cut the chicken into bite-sized cubes. Return the chicken to the skillet, stir, and turn off the heat. Serve over rice or noodles. Garnish with extra parsley, if desired.

meal prep tip:

If you're making this dish for meal prep, make sure you don't overcook the chicken, because it will cook a little more when you reheat it.

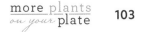

turkey veggie
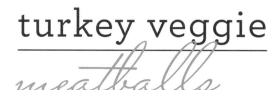
meatballs

YIELD: 4 servings
PREP TIME: 15 minutes
COOK TIME: 20 minutes

These versatile and filling meatballs are full of veggies and full of flavor, and they reheat perfectly. Serve them over zoodles with red pasta sauce, use them to top salads, or pair them with stuffed peppers (page 112) or zucchini boats (page 70). They are practically foolproof; you can adjust the ingredients slightly and still end up with delicious meatballs.

1 pound ground turkey or chicken

1 cup shredded zucchini

1½ cups finely diced bell peppers

1 cup finely diced onions

1 cup chopped mushrooms

4 cloves garlic, minced

1 large egg

2 teaspoons Worcestershire sauce or soy sauce (optional)

¾ cup crushed saltines or soup crackers

1 tablespoon Italian seasoning

1 teaspoon coarse sea salt

1 teaspoon garlic powder

½ teaspoon red pepper flakes

½ teaspoon ground black pepper

1. Preheat the oven to 400°F. Line a rimmed baking sheet with parchment paper and grease the paper lightly with cooking spray.

2. Place all the ingredients in a large bowl and mix with your hands until combined.

3. Using your hands or a small cookie scoop, form the meat mixture into 1- to 1½-inch balls (you should get about 24 meatballs) and arrange them ½ inch apart on the prepared baking sheet; the meatballs can be very close together but should not touch.

4. Bake until browned and bubbling, 18 to 20 minutes. Let the meatballs cool a bit before serving.

meal prep tip:

These meatballs freeze well. I often make a double or triple batch and keep extras in the freezer for when I have zero time to cook.

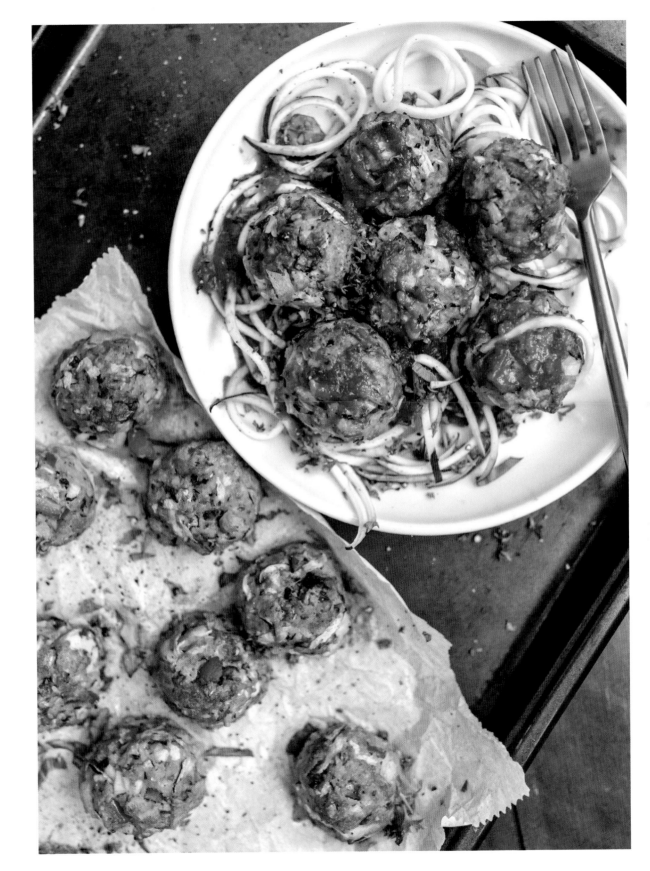

baked
ziti

YIELD: 6 servings
PREP TIME: 15 minutes
COOK TIME: 1 hour

This recipe calls for ground beef or turkey, but you can skip the meat entirely. Although tangy goat cheese is my favorite for this pasta bake, feel free to use any cheese you like, or make the dish vegan by using vegan cream cheese. Be sure to salt the pasta cooking water liberally, as it will season the pasta and reduce the starchiness, helping to spread the sauce more evenly throughout the casserole. Serve the ziti with a salad or the veggies of your choice!

1 pound ziti

3 tablespoons extra-virgin olive oil, divided

1 pound lean ground beef or lean ground turkey

2 cups chopped zucchini

1 cup chopped mushrooms

½ cup diced onions

1½ tablespoons minced garlic

2 (25-ounce) jars red pasta sauce (see notes)

1 tablespoon Italian seasoning

1½ teaspoons dried thyme leaves, crushed

½ teaspoon coarse sea salt

½ teaspoon ground black pepper

3 cups fresh spinach

1 cup crumbled goat cheese

1. Bring a large pot of salted water to a boil. Add the ziti and cook according to the package directions. When done, reserve about 2 cups of the pasta cooking water, then drain the pasta; set aside.

2. Meanwhile, heat 1 tablespoon of the oil in a large skillet or sauté pan over medium-high heat. Once hot, add the ground beef and brown the meat, breaking it up with a spatula as it cooks. Set the meat aside and wipe the pan clean with a paper towel.

3. Add the remaining 2 tablespoons of oil to the skillet. Heat over medium-high heat, then add the chopped zucchini, mushrooms, onions, and garlic and sauté until the veggies have softened a bit and the onions are translucent, about 3 minutes.

4. Pour the red sauce into the skillet with the veggies. Add the Italian seasoning, thyme, salt, and pepper. Use a ladle to fill one of the sauce jars halfway with the reserved pasta water and add that to the skillet to thin the sauce. Fold in the spinach and cook briefly, until wilted.

5. Preheat the oven to 375°F.

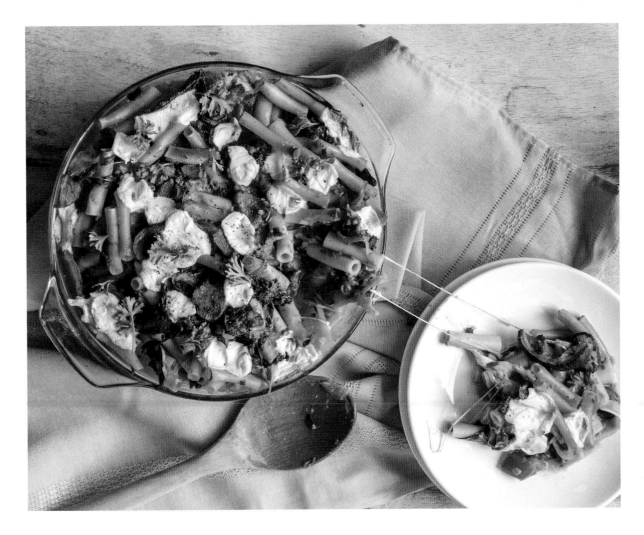

6. Add the drained ziti to the skillet and stir well to ensure it is fully coated with the sauce. Pour the mixture into a 9-inch square or larger baking dish. Stir in most of the goat cheese and crumble the rest on top, then cover the dish with foil. Bake until the sauce is bubbling and the cheese on top is melted, about 45 minutes.

notes: ───────

You may want to add just one and a half jars of pasta sauce if you like your sauce a bit thicker. I prefer mine a little runnier, so I add two full jars. Be sure to cover the dish before baking! It keeps the pasta from drying out.

meal prep tip: ───────

Make this dish in advance to have ready for dinners throughout the week. It will keep in the refrigerator for up to a week or in the freezer for up to 3 months. Just add a tablespoon or two of water to the pasta mixture before reheating it in the microwave to soften the noodles and keep things moist.

chicken

tacos

YIELD: 6 servings
PREP TIME: 15 minutes
COOK TIME: 4 hours

Tacos are a meal I need at least once a month, if not more often, so you will find a few taco recipes in this book. For me, chicken made in a slow cooker always tastes way better. You can make the chicken filling on a rimmed baking sheet in the oven if you prefer, or you can really cut down on the prep time and buy a precooked rotisserie chicken. Just sauté the onions and bell peppers in some olive oil until softened, then put the remaining ingredients for the filling in a saucepan and heat them up.

CHICKEN FILLING:

1½ pounds boneless, skinless chicken breasts

1 cup sliced onions

1 cup chopped bell peppers (green or red)

½ (4-ounce) can diced green chilies (about ¼ cup)

½ cup low-sodium chicken broth

1½ teaspoons chili powder

1 teaspoon garlic powder

1 teaspoon onion powder

1 teaspoon paprika

½ teaspoon chipotle powder

½ teaspoon ground cumin

½ teaspoon coarse sea salt

1½ cups frozen corn kernels

½ cup salsa

FOR SERVING:

Small flour or corn tortillas

Sliced or diced avocado

Halved cherry tomatoes

Fresh cilantro leaves

Put all the ingredients for the chicken filling, except for the corn and salsa, in a 6-quart slow cooker and cook on high for 3 to 4 hours or on low for 6 to 8 hours, until the chicken is tender. Use two forks to shred the chicken in the slow cooker, then stir in the corn and salsa. Cover, turn the slow cooker to high, and heat just until the corn is warmed. To serve, fill the tortillas with the chicken mixture and top with avocado, tomatoes, and cilantro.

meal prep tip:

Divide the chicken filling among single-serving containers and store in the refrigerator for up to 4 days; reheat in the microwave. Store the tortillas and fresh toppings separately and assemble the tacos just before you eat them.

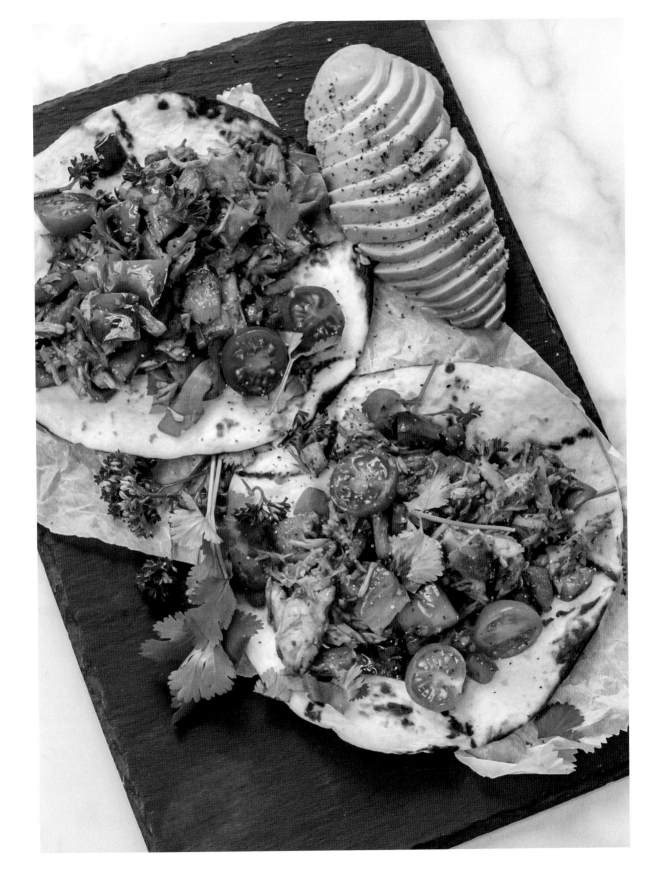

sneaky turkey
meatloaf

YIELD: 4 servings
PREP TIME: 10 minutes
COOK TIME: 45 minutes

I have been making this meatloaf for years. My recipe has evolved over time, and it just keeps getting better! It has a lot of sneaky veggies in it; your family will not even notice how they've been mixed right into this comforting meal. Pair the meatloaf with steamed broccoli, roasted potatoes, the roasted veggies from the Harvest Salad (page 154), or Sweet Potato Fries with Parmesan (page 162).

1 pound lean ground turkey

1¼ cups shredded zucchini

1 cup diced fire-roasted tomatoes

1 cup old-fashioned oats or plain breadcrumbs

4 cloves garlic, minced

1 large egg

2 teaspoons Worcestershire sauce or soy sauce

1 teaspoon ground dried oregano

1 teaspoon dried thyme leaves

½ teaspoon paprika

½ teaspoon coarse sea salt

½ teaspoon ground black pepper

1½ teaspoons Worcestershire sauce or soy sauce

1½ tablespoons brown sugar

¼ teaspoon ground nutmeg

GLAZE (OPTIONAL):

½ cup ketchup

1 tablespoon prepared yellow mustard

1. Preheat the oven to 375°F. Line an 8½ by 4½-inch loaf pan with parchment paper, leaving some overhanging for easy removal.

2. Put all the meatloaf ingredients in a large bowl and mix well with your hands. Transfer the mixture to the prepared pan.

3. In a small bowl, whisk together all the ingredients for the glaze, if using. Pour the glaze evenly over the meatloaf.

4. Bake for 45 minutes, until the top is lightly browned and the juices run clear when pricked in the center with a fork (or when the temperature in the center reaches 165°F). Let the loaf rest for about 5 minutes to set, then remove from the pan; slice and serve.

meal prep tip:

This recipe is great for meal prep. You can store the meatloaf in the refrigerator for up to 4 days or freezer for up to 3 months. You can also make sandwiches with the leftovers if you need to change things up!

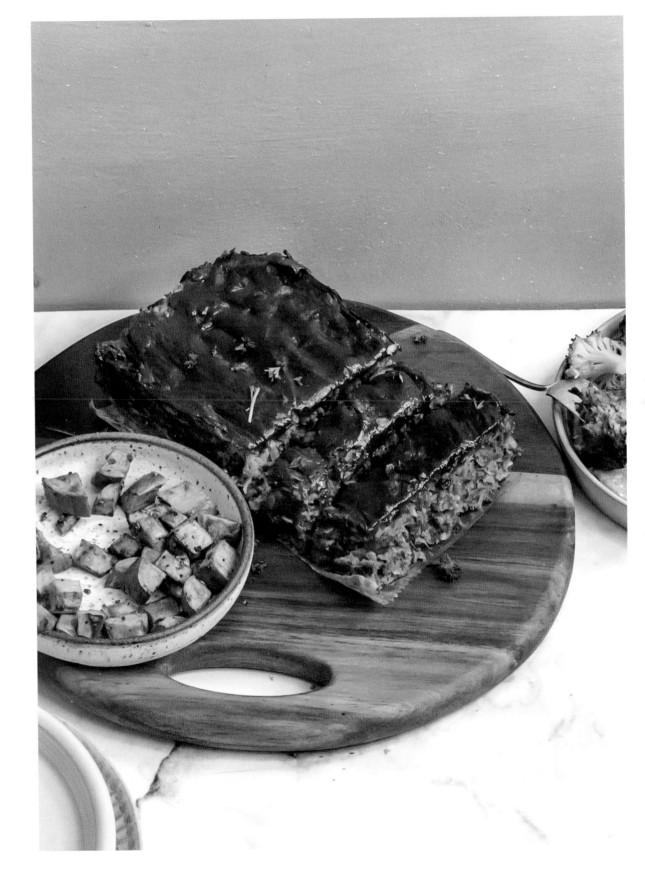

stuffed

peppers

YIELD: 8 servings

PREP TIME: 15 minutes (not including time to cook quinoa)

COOK TIME: 40 minutes

Have you ever tried stuffed peppers? If not, you've been missing out on an easy way to get more plants on your plate. Bell peppers are the perfect vehicle to hold more veggies, meats, and seasonings. I love making stuffed peppers when I want more veggies and fiber in my diet. They are filling, too. You can make this meal totally plant-based by skipping the ground turkey; it will be just as delicious. The cheese helps bind the filling mixture together, but I often make this dish without the cheese.

4 large bell peppers (any color)

2 tablespoons extra-virgin olive oil

1 pound ground turkey

½ cup shredded carrots

½ cup diced mushrooms

¼ cup diced onions

1 tablespoon plus 1 teaspoon roughly chopped fresh parsley, divided

1½ teaspoons Italian seasoning

1 teaspoon garlic powder

½ teaspoon chili powder

¼ teaspoon ground black pepper

¼ teaspoon coarse sea salt

1 (15-ounce) can diced fire-roasted tomatoes

1½ cups cooked quinoa

1 cup shredded mozzarella cheese or vegan mozzarella, plus extra for topping (optional)

1. Preheat the oven to 375°F. Grease a 13 by 9-inch baking dish (or a casserole dish large enough to hold all eight pepper halves) with cooking oil spray.

2. Slice the peppers in half lengthwise. Remove and discard the stems and seeds. Arrange the peppers in the prepared baking dish with the cut sides facing up.

3. Heat the oil in a large nonstick skillet over medium-high heat. Add the ground turkey, carrots, mushrooms, onions, 1 teaspoon of the parsley, the spices, and salt. Cook, crumbling the meat with a wooden spoon, until the turkey is fully browned and cooked through and the vegetables are tender, about 4 minutes.

4. Drain any excess liquid, then add the diced tomatoes and quinoa and stir to combine. Let the juice boil down a bit. Stir in the cheese, if using.

5. Scoop the meat and veggie mixture into the pepper halves. Sprinkle with extra cheese, if desired. Bake until the peppers are tender, 30 to 35 minutes. Garnish with the remaining tablespoon of fresh parsley and enjoy!

meal prep tip:

These stuffed peppers will keep in the refrigerator for up to 4 days, or you can freeze them for up to 3 months.

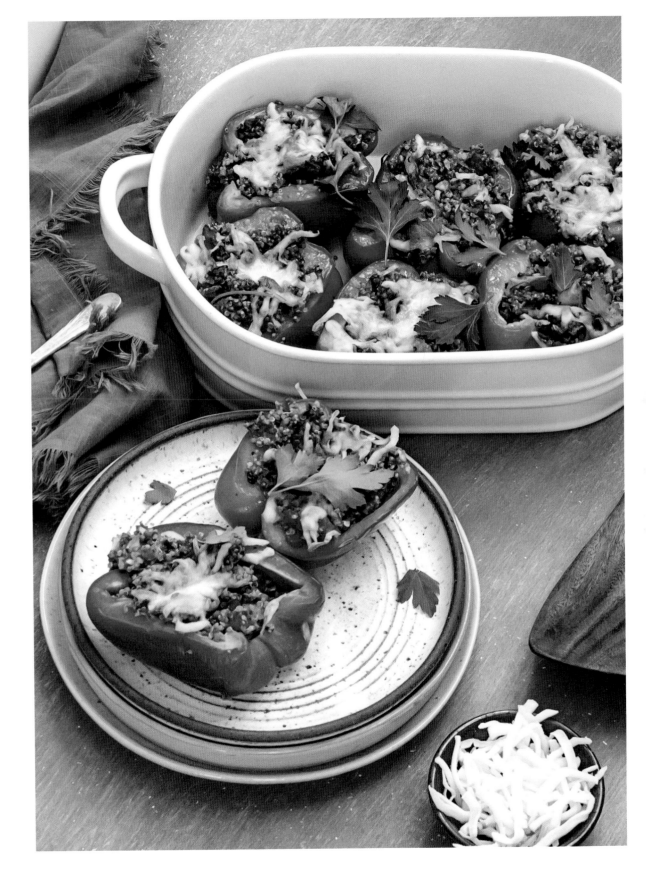

three-bean
turkey chili

YIELD: 6 to 8 servings
PREP TIME: 10 minutes
COOK TIME: 1 hour 10 minutes or 5 hours, depending on cooking method

I grew up making this chili with my mom, and over time I have made it more of my own by adding veggies to it. We love this flavorful chili throughout the fall and winter months—it is so much healthier than your average chili. To make the recipe entirely plant-based, omit the turkey and add another can of black beans. I've given you the option of making the chili on the stovetop or in a slow cooker, which I find yields a much more flavorful chili.

1 pound ground turkey

1 tablespoon extra-virgin olive oil

1 cup chopped onions

2 teaspoons minced garlic

2 (15.5-ounce) cans light red kidney beans, drained and rinsed

2 (15.5-ounce) cans dark red kidney beans, drained and rinsed

1 (15.5-ounce) can black beans, drained and rinsed

1 (28-ounce) can peeled whole Italian-style tomatoes, cut up

1 (14.5-ounce) can stewed tomatoes

2 (4-ounce) cans diced green chilies

1 jalapeño pepper, chopped (optional)

2 cups chopped zucchini (about 3 medium zucchinis)

1 (8-ounce) package sliced mushrooms

⅓ cup chili powder

1 teaspoon ground dried oregano

1 teaspoon coarse sea salt

¼ teaspoon red pepper flakes (optional)

2 cups water

TOPPINGS:

Chopped fresh cilantro

Crushed tortilla chips

Sliced jalapeño peppers

Sliced radishes

1. **If using a slow cooker,** crumble the ground turkey into the slow cooker and stir in the remaining ingredients. Cook on high for 4 hours or on low for 8 hours. Stir well, then cook for 1 hour longer, or until everything is tender.

   If using the stovetop, heat the oil in a Dutch oven or soup pot over medium heat. Add the onions and garlic and cook, stirring frequently, until the onions are translucent, about 3 minutes. Add the ground turkey and cook, crumbling the meat with a wooden spoon, until lightly browned, about 4 minutes. Add the remaining ingredients in the order listed. Simmer over low heat, uncovered, for 1 hour, until the beans and veggies are tender.

2. Top the chili with cilantro, tortilla chips, jalapeños, and radishes and serve.

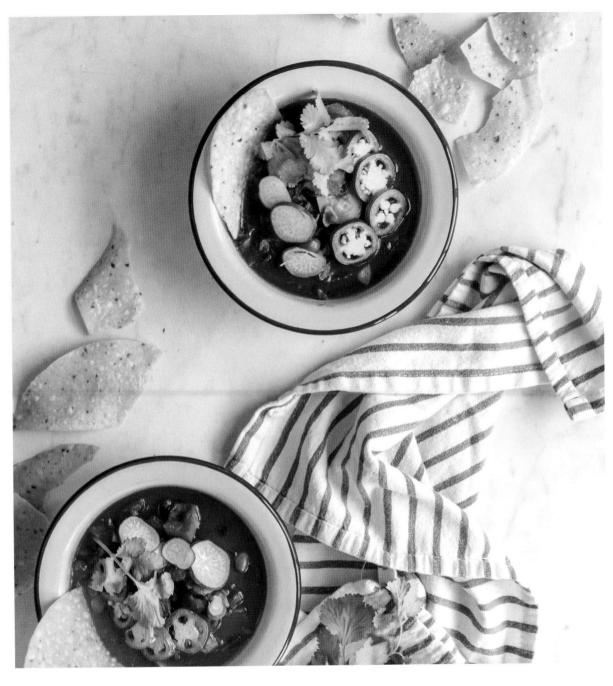

meal prep tip:

If meal prepping the chili, allow it to cool completely, then transfer it to glass containers and store in the refrigerator for up to 4 days. To freeze it, transfer it to a resealable plastic bag and freeze for up to 3 months.

turkey feta meatballs
with red pepper sauce

YIELD: 4 servings
PREP TIME: 10 minutes
COOK TIME: 40 minutes

This is one of my favorite recipes in the entire book! It's a versatile dish that can be paired with roasted veggies, sliced avocado, and so many other foods. I like to serve these meatballs over rice or salad greens.

MEATBALLS:

1 pound ground turkey

1 cup crumbled feta cheese

½ cup old-fashioned oats

½ cup chopped fresh spinach

½ cup finely chopped red onions

1 tablespoon chopped fresh cilantro

1 tablespoon ground dried oregano

1 tablespoon chopped fresh parsley

1½ teaspoons minced garlic

½ teaspoon dried marjoram leaves

½ teaspoon dried thyme leaves

¼ teaspoon coarse sea salt

¼ teaspoon ground black pepper

1 large egg yolk

RED PEPPER SAUCE:

¼ cup tahini, stirred well

⅓ cup roasted red peppers, jarred or homemade (see page 96)

¼ cup warm water

1½ teaspoons honey

1½ teaspoons fresh squeezed lemon juice

1½ teaspoons garlic powder

¼ teaspoon coarse sea salt

1. Preheat the oven to 375°F. Line a rimmed baking sheet with parchment paper.

2. Put all the ingredients for the meatballs in a big bowl and mix using your hands. Really work the feta into the mixture. Roll into 1-inch balls and place on the prepared baking sheet. Bake for 30 to 40 minutes, until browned on the outside and cooked through.

3. While the meatballs are baking, make the sauce: Put all the ingredients in a medium bowl (if using an immersion blender) or in a blender and blend until smooth.

4. Serve the meatballs topped with the sauce.

meal prep tip:

You can change up this dish throughout the week. Grab any veggies you have in the fridge and roast them up to round out your meal; I especially like red bell peppers and cauliflower or broccoli. This recipe is also easy to double; you can freeze the extra meatballs to reheat later. The red pepper sauce also makes a nice salad dressing.

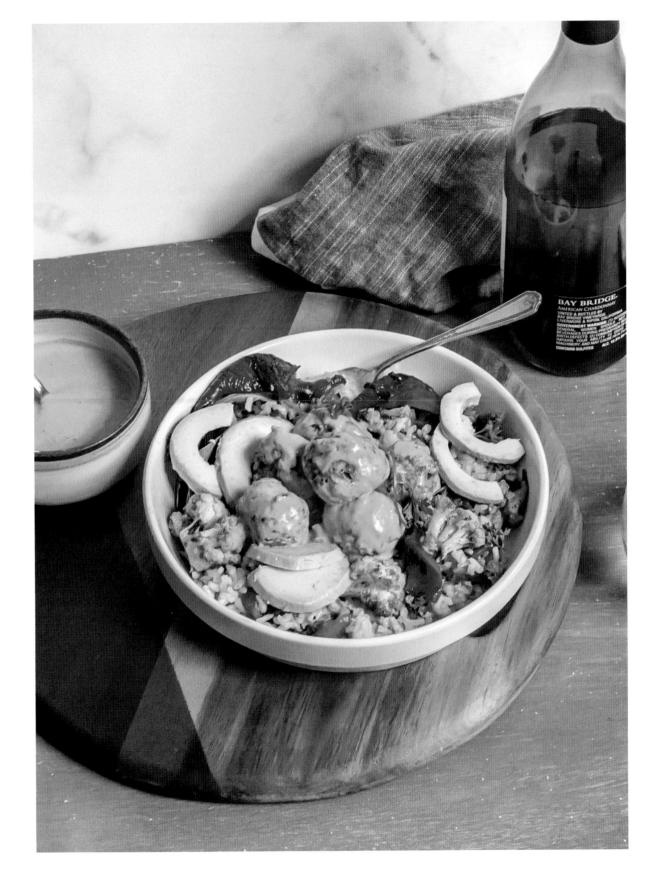

chicken & veggie
sheet pan meal

YIELD: 4 servings
PREP TIME: 10 minutes
COOK TIME: 25 minutes

This dish was invented by my husband, Matt, who loves to throw together new meals. Because Matt often does the dishes, he tries to dirty as few as possible when he cooks—something we all can appreciate! Sheet pan meals are the best for easy cleanup. You can pair this dish with any veggie rice, or add it to a bed of fresh greens and have yourself a delicious salad. I highly recommend making my Plant-Based Ranch Dressing (page 156) and drizzling it over everything before serving. The red pepper sauce on page 116 would also be tasty.

2 to 3 boneless, skinless chicken breasts (about 1½ pounds), cut into bite-sized pieces

2 cups chopped broccoli

1 cup chopped yellow squash

1 medium red onion, chopped

½ cup grape tomatoes

¼ cup fresh squeezed lime juice

1 teaspoon garlic powder

1 teaspoon paprika

1 teaspoon dried rosemary leaves

1 teaspoon dried thyme leaves

½ teaspoon coarse sea salt

½ teaspoon ground black pepper

½ teaspoon red pepper flakes (optional)

2 tablespoons extra-virgin olive oil

1. Preheat the oven to 450°F. Line a rimmed baking sheet with parchment paper.

2. Put all the ingredients except the oil in a large bowl. Mix well to ensure that the chicken and veggies are evenly coated with the seasonings. Spread the mixture in an even layer on the prepared baking sheet, spreading out the pieces as much as you can. Drizzle the oil over everything.

3. Bake until the chicken is cooked all the way through (the internal temperature should reach 165°F) and the veggies are tender, 20 to 25 minutes, and enjoy!

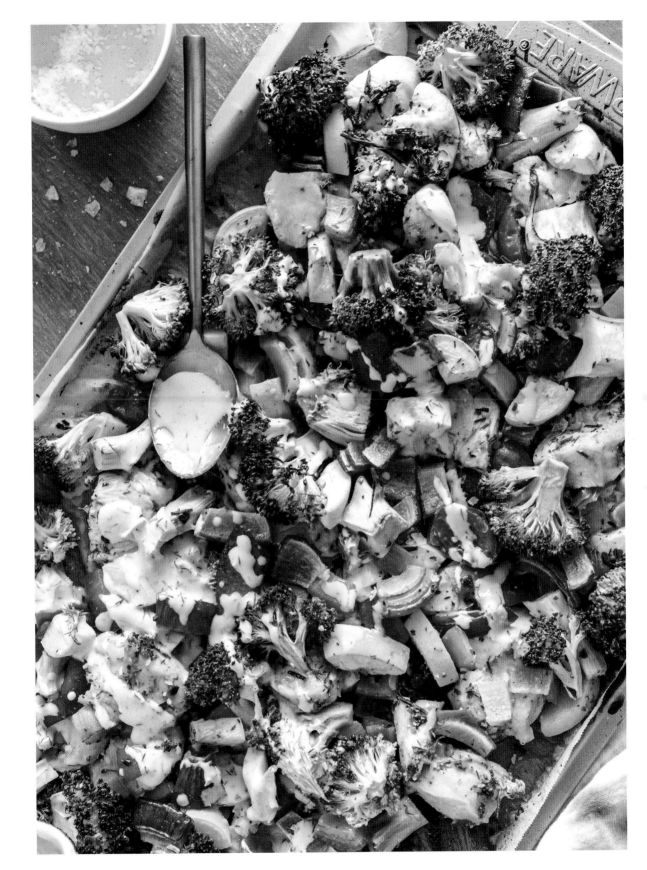

shredded bbq chicken
& peppers

YIELD: 4 servings
PREP TIME: 10 minutes
COOK TIME: 4 hours

Nothing is better than a slow cooker meal with few steps and little mess! This recipe is great when you want a healthier comfort meal with lots of options for customization. You can pile the chicken mixture over lettuce and have a salad, eat it over rice, or use it as a taco filling. The choice is yours, and trust me when I say that the whole family will love it. This is another husband-approved meal; he requests it year-round.

3 cups chopped green bell peppers

1 cup chopped onions

2 tablespoons minced garlic

2 cups BBQ sauce

½ cup low-sodium chicken broth or water

2 tablespoons medium-hot hot sauce, such as Frank's RedHot (optional)

2 teaspoons smoked paprika

2 teaspoons liquid smoke

1 to 1½ pounds boneless, skinless chicken breasts

2 cups cooked rice, or 4 to 6 cups chopped spinach or romaine lettuce, for serving

Red pepper flakes, for garnish (optional)

1. Put the peppers, onions, garlic, BBQ sauce, broth, hot sauce (if using), smoked paprika, and liquid smoke in a medium bowl and mix well. Place the chicken breasts in a 6-quart slow cooker and pour the sauce over the chicken. Cook on high for about 4 hours or on low for about 8 hours, until the chicken is fork-tender.

2. Remove the breasts from the slow cooker and use two forks to gently shred the chicken. Return the chicken to the slow cooker to heat through. Serve the chicken, peppers, and sauce over the rice or greens, garnished with red pepper flakes, if desired.

meal prep tip:

This dish is great for meal prep; it reheats beautifully, and you can change it up throughout the week. If meal prepping this dish, separate the rice into containers and top it with the shredded chicken. Instead of serving the leftovers over rice or lettuce as suggested here, feel free to turn it into a shredded chicken sandwich.

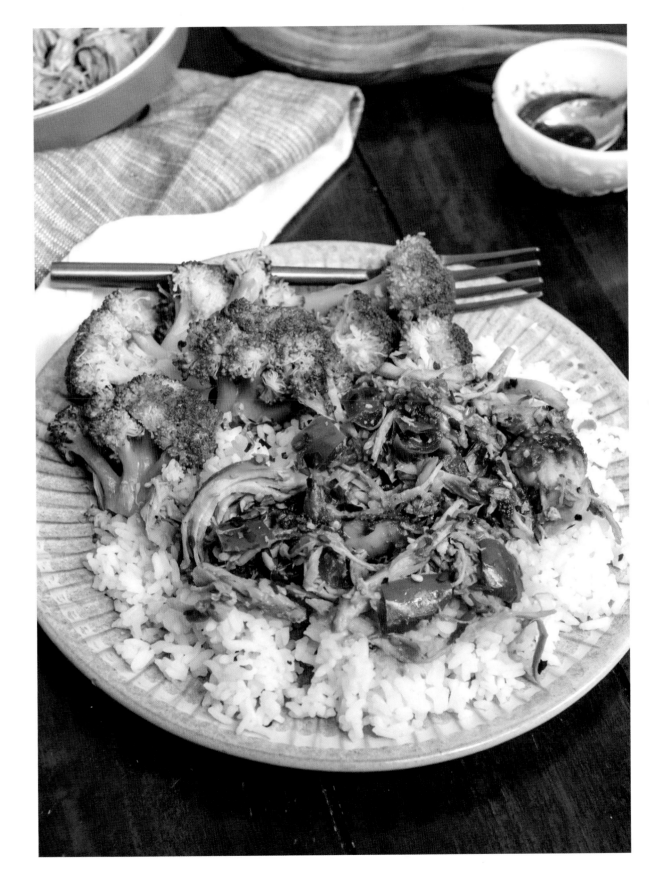

almond cashew coconut
chicken tenders
with honey mustard

YIELD: 4 servings
PREP TIME: 10 minutes
COOK TIME: 18 minutes

Chicken tenders are my favorite way to enjoy chicken, and my favorite sauce to serve them with is honey mustard. These chicken tenders take me back to my childhood, and they are easy to make. Pair them with Sweet Potato Fries with Parmesan (page 162) or steamed broccoli. Some RightRice would be a nutritious companion as well.

½ cup raw almonds

½ cup raw cashews

½ cup unsweetened shredded coconut

1 teaspoon garlic powder

1 teaspoon onion powder

½ teaspoon coarse sea salt

½ teaspoon red pepper flakes (optional)

2 large eggs

2 tablespoons water

1 teaspoon coconut aminos or soy sauce

1 pound boneless, skinless chicken breasts

HONEY MUSTARD:

3 tablespoons Dijon mustard

1½ tablespoons water

1 teaspoon honey

1. Preheat the oven to 350°F. Line a rimmed baking sheet with parchment paper.

2. In a food processor, pulse the almonds, cashews, shredded coconut, garlic powder, onion powder, salt, and red pepper flakes, if using, until the mixture has a crumbly consistency. Transfer to a shallow bowl or plate.

3. In a medium bowl, whisk together the eggs, water, and aminos. Cut the chicken breasts into 3- to 4-inch tenders. Pat dry with a paper towel. Dip a tender in the egg wash, then in the nut mixture. Be sure to cover the entire tender. Lay the tender flat on the prepared baking sheet and repeat with the remaining chicken, egg wash, and nut mixture.

4. Bake until the chicken is opaque all the way through in the thickest part, 16 to 18 minutes.

5. Meanwhile, make the honey mustard: In a small dipping bowl, whisk together the mustard, water, and honey. Add more water or mustard to get the desired consistency.

6. Serve the chicken tenders with the honey mustard.

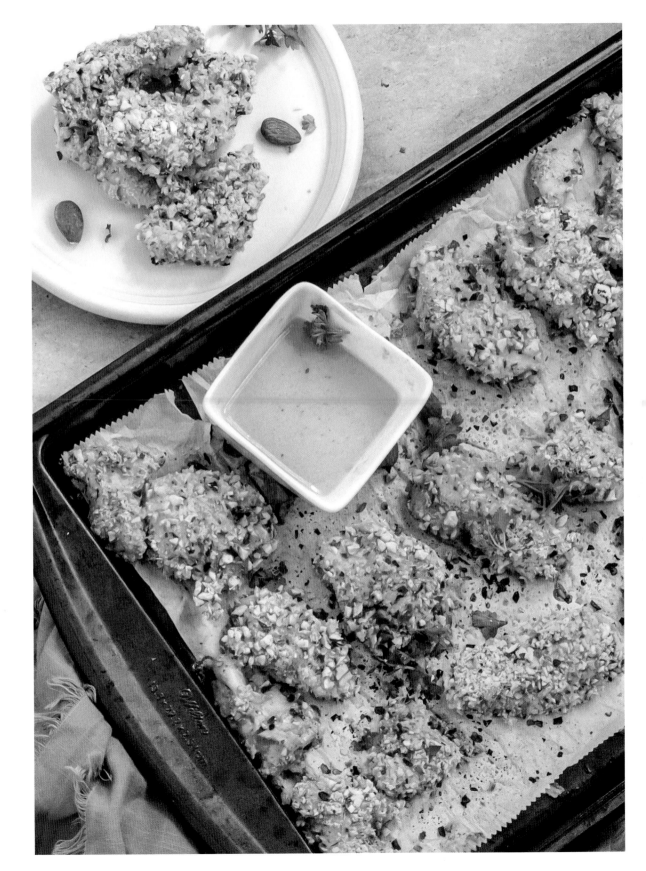

chicken sausage
fajitas

YIELD: 4 servings
PREP TIME: 10 minutes
COOK TIME: 18 minutes

Craving fajitas from your favorite Mexican joint? Make them fresh at home instead! This recipe has less grease and fewer calories and tastes just as good (if not better!) than your local Mexican restaurant's version. The fajita mixture can be served with tortillas or romaine lettuce leaves, or over chopped greens for a hearty salad.

3 tablespoons extra-virgin olive oil

4 cups sliced bell peppers (any color)

1½ cups sliced red or yellow onions

1 cup diced zucchini

4 cloves garlic, minced

1½ teaspoons liquid smoke

1½ tablespoons chili powder

1½ teaspoons paprika

½ teaspoon ground cumin

½ teaspoon ground dried marjoram

½ teaspoon ground dried oregano

½ teaspoon coarse sea salt

1 pound precooked chicken sausages, sliced into coins

Flour tortillas or romaine lettuce leaves, for serving

OPTIONAL TOPPINGS:

Sour cream

Sliced avocado

1. Heat the oil in a large skillet or sauté pan over medium-high heat. Add the bell peppers and onions and sauté for a few minutes, until starting to sweat. Add the zucchini, garlic, liquid smoke, chili powder, paprika, cumin, marjoram, oregano, and salt. Continue to sauté until the peppers and onions are slightly charred, another 8 to 10 minutes.

2. Add the sausage slices and sauté until browned and heated through, 3 to 5 minutes.

3. Serve the sausage, peppers, and onions on tortillas or lettuce leaves, topped with sour cream and/or avocado slices, if desired.

meal prep tip:

You can meal prep this dish in advance and serve it all week. The fajita mixture keeps really well in the fridge.

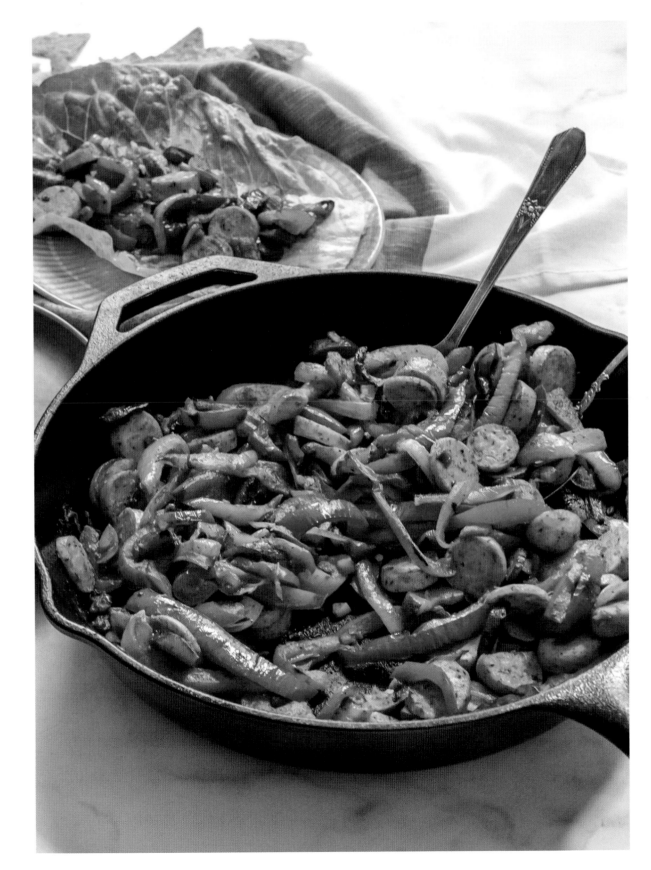

pepperoni
rigatoni

YIELD: 4 servings
PREP TIME: 10 minutes
COOK TIME: 25 minutes

Two friends introduced me to this dish in my early twenties. We came home after a day of snowboarding, and they had this pasta dish in the fridge for lunch. Unfortunately, I lost the recipe they wrote down for me, so I had to make my own version. I love how this dish gets better and better as the week goes on.

You can use traditional pepperoni, turkey pepperoni, or plant-based pepperoni. Whichever you choose, you will love this dish!

8 ounces rigatoni

1 tablespoon extra-virgin olive oil

1 cup chopped yellow squash

½ cup chopped roasted red peppers, jarred or homemade (see page 96)

3 cloves garlic, minced

2 jalapeño peppers, chopped

1 (32-ounce) jar red pasta sauce

½ teaspoon Italian seasoning

¼ teaspoon onion powder

1 cup sliced pepperoni

1 (14.5-ounce) can low-sodium chicken broth

Coarse sea salt (if needed)

Thinly sliced fresh basil leaves, for garnish (optional)

1. Cook the pasta in a pot of salted water according to the package directions. When done, drain and set aside.

2. Meanwhile, prepare the sauce: Heat the oil in a Dutch oven over medium heat. Add the squash, roasted red peppers, garlic, and jalapeños and cook, stirring often, for 5 to 8 minutes, until the veggies are starting to sweat. Add the red sauce, Italian seasoning, and onion powder and simmer for about 5 minutes to allow the flavors to meld.

3. Add the pepperoni and chicken broth; simmer over low heat for another 10 to 15 minutes to release the pepperoni flavors into the sauce. Taste and season with salt if needed. Stir in the rigatoni, garnish with fresh basil, if desired, and serve!

meal prep tip:
Cook the pasta in advance to make this dish come together even more quickly!

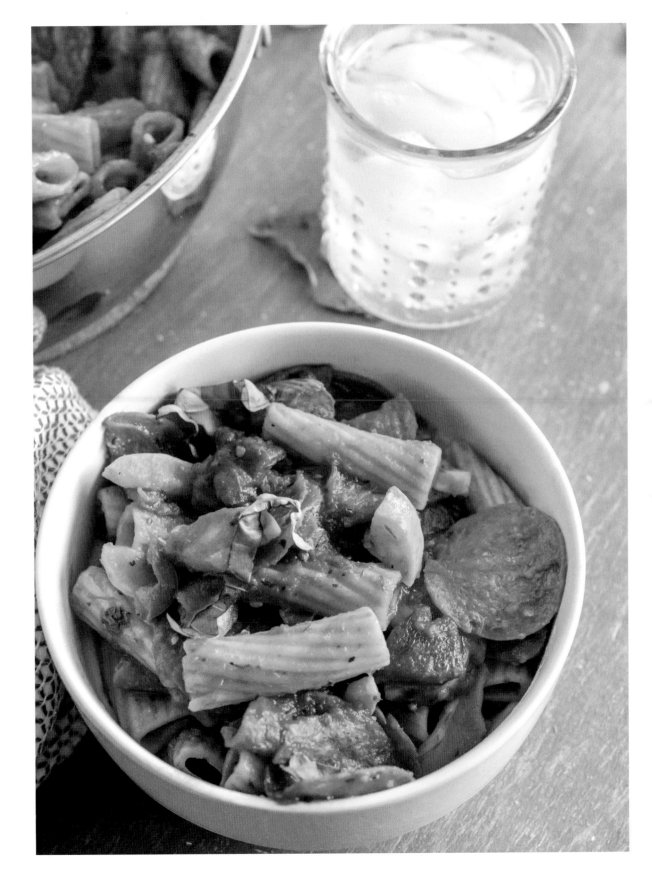

beef spaghetti squash
with tzatziki

YIELD: 4 servings
PREP TIME: 15 minutes
COOK TIME: 30 minutes

This was my family's favorite dish to taste-test during the writing of this cookbook, and they've been requesting it ever since. It is a comforting meal that won't leave you feeling weighed down. To make it totally plant-based, skip the ground beef and increase the amount of each vegetable by 1 cup. You can also use crumbled tempeh in place of the ground beef in this recipe.

1 medium spaghetti squash

1 pound lean ground beef

1 cup diced red bell peppers

½ cup diced red onions

1 cup chopped mushrooms

1 cup chopped fresh spinach

3 cloves garlic, minced

1 teaspoon dried ground marjoram

1 teaspoon dried ground oregano leaves

1 teaspoon dried ground thyme leaves

½ teaspoon coarse sea salt

½ teaspoon ground black pepper

TZATZIKI:

½ cup plant-based sour cream or plain Greek yogurt

3 tablespoons tahini, stirred well

3 tablespoons shredded cucumber, liquid squeezed out

2 cloves garlic, minced

2 tablespoons water

1 teaspoon fresh dill

½ teaspoon fresh squeezed lemon juice

½ teaspoon coarse sea salt

¼ teaspoon ground black pepper

1. Preheat the oven to 400°F. Line a rimmed baking sheet with aluminum foil.

2. Using a sharp paring knife, prick the squash all over. Place the squash on the prepared baking sheet and bake until soft enough to pierce with a fork, about 30 minutes. When done, cut the squash in half lengthwise and remove the seeds. Optionally, use the fork to scrape the squash strings into a large bowl. (Keep the strings in the shells if you'd like to present the dish that way. Note that taking the squash out of the shells will stretch the meal further; 1½ cups of squash per serving is plenty.)

3. Meanwhile, brown the beef in a large skillet or sauté pan over medium heat, breaking it up into crumbles, about 5 minutes. Add the bell peppers and onions and cook, stirring often, until slightly softened, about 5 minutes, then add the mushrooms and spinach and cook until those have softened, another 5 minutes.

4. Add the garlic, herbs, salt, and pepper; mix well. Cook until everything is nicely blended and softened, another 5 to 10 minutes. Remove the pan from the heat and set it aside while you make the tzatziki.

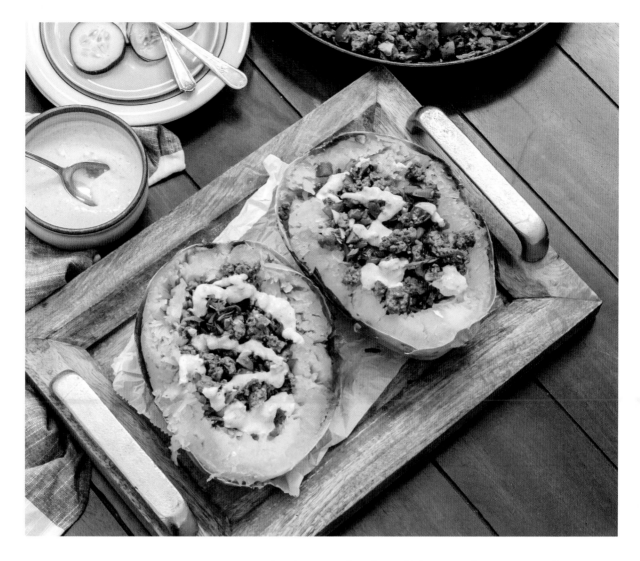

5. Make the tzatziki: Place all the ingredients in a medium bowl and blend with an immersion blender until smooth, or use a food processor or high-powered blender.

6. Spoon the beef and veggie mixture over the squash "noodles" and serve with a generous drizzle of the tzatziki on top.

meal prep tip: ———————————

This is a perfect recipe to meal prep for the week, and it's easy to stretch with more veggies. Just add ½ cup or more of each additional veggie to the mix and double the seasonings.

turkey veggie
tacos

YIELD: 4 servings
PREP TIME: 10 minutes
COOK TIME: 15 minutes

These tacos have been a staple in my house for years; I cannot get enough of them. Regardless of whether you use ground turkey or a meat substitute, the tacos will be tasty because they're packed with vegetables and spices. This recipe was inspired by the beef tacos that my mom would make for us growing up. I have since made them "lighter," full of veggies and with cleaner ingredients.

2 tablespoons extra-virgin olive oil

1 pound lean ground turkey

1½ cups chopped zucchini or yellow squash (about 2 medium squash)

1 cup chopped mushrooms

1 cup diced onions

4 cloves garlic, minced

1½ tablespoons chili powder

1½ teaspoons paprika

1 teaspoon ground dried oregano

½ teaspoon ground cumin

½ teaspoon garlic powder

⅛ teaspoon cayenne pepper

½ teaspoon coarse sea salt

FOR SERVING:

Small corn or flour tortillas, or chopped romaine lettuce or mixed greens

Fresh cilantro leaves

Halved grape tomatoes

Sliced avocado

Sliced jalapeños

Sour cream

Cashew Queso (page 214)

1. Heat the oil in a large skillet or sauté pan over medium-high heat. When hot, add the ground turkey; cook, breaking up the meat into crumbles, until it is starting to brown, about 4 minutes.

2. Add the zucchini, mushrooms, onions, garlic, spices, and salt. Sauté until the veggies are softened, about 10 minutes.

3. Serve the turkey and veggie filling in tortillas or on a bed of greens with your favorite taco toppings.

meal prep tip:

This is a great recipe to meal prep for the week, and it's easy to double and/or to stretch with extra veggies. I like to add the taco filling to fresh salad greens to make a taco salad bowl.

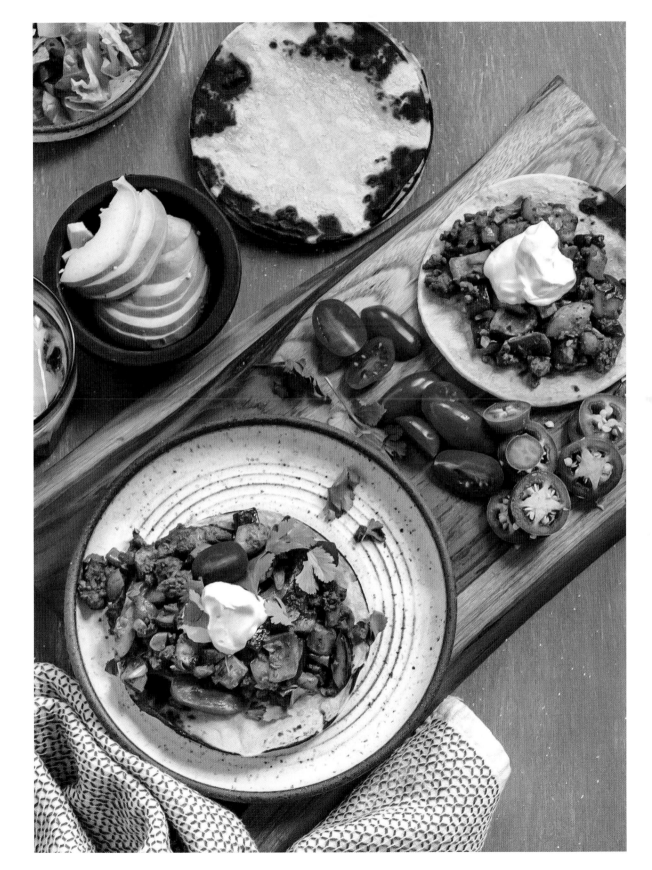

date night recipes

I wanted the recipes in this chapter to be a little more romantic. These dishes are still packed with vegetables; they're just as nutritious and tasty as the other recipes in the book. However, these dishes take a little more effort to prepare, and most of them are best eaten fresh. You can share them with your partner or a friend or have a few servings all to yourself.

These recipes are close to my heart. I have been making them with my husband, Matt, for years, and I am excited to share them with the world.

You can also use these recipes to vary your weekly meal plan. If you're feeling burnout from leftovers, make yourself a nice fresh dinner with a bottle of wine midweek to switch things up—no one is judging you!

Maple Bourbon Salmon with Veggie Rice & Broccoli | 133

Pan-Fried Chicken & Veggies with Rosemary Gravy | 136

Mediterranean Red Pepper Risotto with Shrimp | 138

Mushroom & Brussels Sprouts Pizza | 140

Sunday Burgers | 142

Sweet Potato Tacos | 144

Plant-Based Tuscan Alfredo with Artichokes & Mushrooms | 146

Teriyaki Salmon Sheet Pan Dinner | 148

maple bourbon salmon
with veggie rice & broccoli

YIELD: 2 servings
PREP TIME: 10 minutes (not including time to cook rice)
COOK TIME: 30 minutes

This restaurant-quality dish is quite an upgrade from the typical weeknight meal, especially when served with wine or whiskey. Bonus points if you eat in your pajamas! You can substitute chicken, tofu, or portobello mushroom caps for the salmon and have an equally delicious meal; see the tip on page 135.

MAPLE BOURBON GLAZE:

½ cup bourbon

¼ cup maple syrup

1½ teaspoons Dijon mustard

½ teaspoon chipotle powder

½ teaspoon garlic powder

2 tablespoons extra-virgin olive oil, divided

3 cups broccoli florets

1 cup sliced mushrooms

½ teaspoon coarse sea salt

¼ teaspoon ground black pepper

½ teaspoon chipotle powder

2 (8-ounce) skin-on salmon fillets

1 cup cooked RightRice or other type of veggie rice, for serving

1. Make the glaze: Combine the bourbon, maple syrup, mustard, chipotle powder, and garlic powder in a small saucepan. Simmer over low heat until thickened, 15 to 20 minutes. Remove from the heat and set aside.

2. When the glaze has about 10 minutes left to simmer, heat 1 tablespoon of the oil in a large skillet or sauté pan over medium-high heat. When hot, add the broccoli and mushrooms. Season with the salt, pepper, and chipotle powder. Sauté for 8 to 10 minutes, until the broccoli has a little char on it but is bright green. Transfer to a plate and set aside.

3. Wipe the skillet clean and put it back over medium-high heat. Pour in the remaining 1 tablespoon of oil. Place the salmon skin side down in the pan. Brush the top of the salmon with a thin layer of the glaze and cook for 6 to 7 minutes. Some glaze will fall around the salmon and may burn a bit, but the salmon itself will be fine. Add another ½ tablespoon of oil to the pan, if needed.

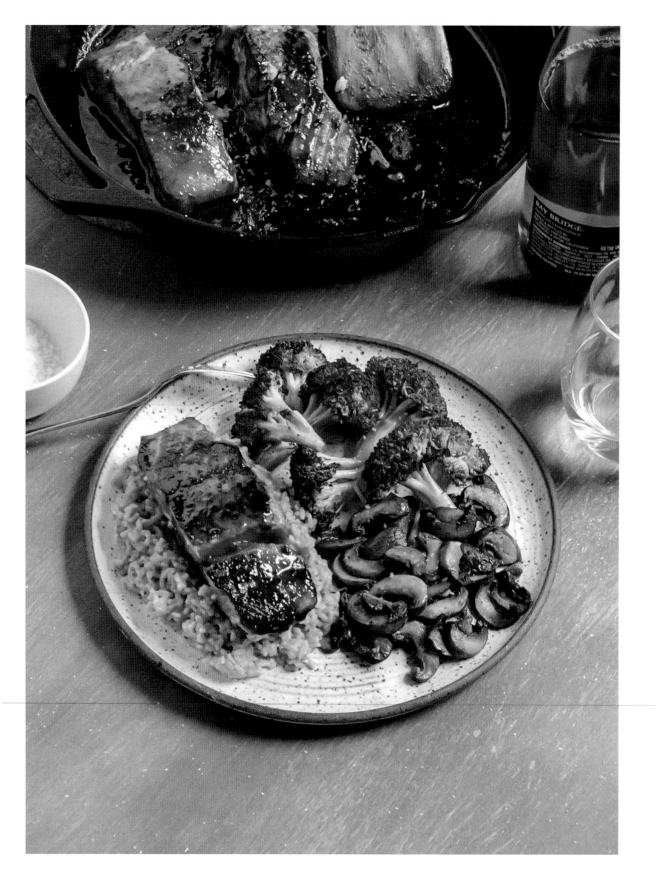

4. Flip the salmon and cook until the fish flakes easily, 3 to 4 minutes. Use a pair of tongs to carefully peel the skin off and brush more glaze on the exposed salmon flesh, reserving some of the glaze for the vegetables. Take the salmon off the heat.

5. Serve with the prepared vegetables and rice on the side, drizzled with leftover glaze.

meal prep tip:

If making this dish with chicken, cubed firm or extra-firm tofu, or portobello mushroom caps, bake at 375°F for 10 minutes. Brush with the glaze a few times. Continue to bake for 10 more minutes. Remove from the oven and brush with another layer of the glaze before serving.

pan-fried chicken & veggies
with rosemary gravy

YIELD: 2 servings

PREP TIME: 15 minutes (not including time to cook rice)

COOK TIME: 35 minutes

This recipe was an experiment that went over very well. The gravy is light and fragrant of fresh rosemary and won't make you feel heavy. It makes enough for leftovers the next day, too. You can easily substitute tofu or portobello mushroom caps to make this dish entirely plant-based.

1½ teaspoons extra-virgin olive oil

2 (6-ounce) boneless, skinless chicken breasts

¼ teaspoon coarse sea salt

¼ teaspoon ground black pepper

¼ teaspoon garlic powder

ROSEMARY GRAVY:

1½ teaspoons extra-virgin olive oil

1½ teaspoons all-purpose flour

¾ cup So Delicious Original coconut milk creamer or SILK unsweetened almond milk

1½ teaspoons chopped fresh rosemary

¾ cup chopped zucchini

½ teaspoon vegetable bouillon paste

¾ cup chopped fresh spinach

½ cup grape tomatoes

1 tablespoon fresh squeezed lemon juice

1 cup cooked RightRice or other type of veggie rice, for serving (optional)

1. Heat the oil in a medium skillet or sauté pan over medium-high heat. When hot, season the chicken breasts with the salt and pepper and cook them until browned on one side, about 10 minutes. Flip the chicken, lower the heat a bit, and cook for another 10 minutes, or until no longer pink in the center. Remove the pan from the heat, then transfer the chicken to a plate and set aside. Wipe the skillet clean.

2. Make the gravy: Heat the oil in the same skillet over medium heat. Quickly whisk in the flour. Add the creamer and continue to whisk briskly while adding the rosemary. Continue cooking until the gravy has browned slightly, about 5 minutes.

3. Add the zucchini and bouillon paste. Simmer, stirring occasionally, for about 5 minutes to soften the zucchini. Then add the spinach and tomatoes; mix well.

4. Return the chicken breasts to the skillet, cover with a lid, and simmer to rewarm the chicken, about 5 minutes. Squeeze the lemon juice over the chicken and gravy and serve over rice, if desired.

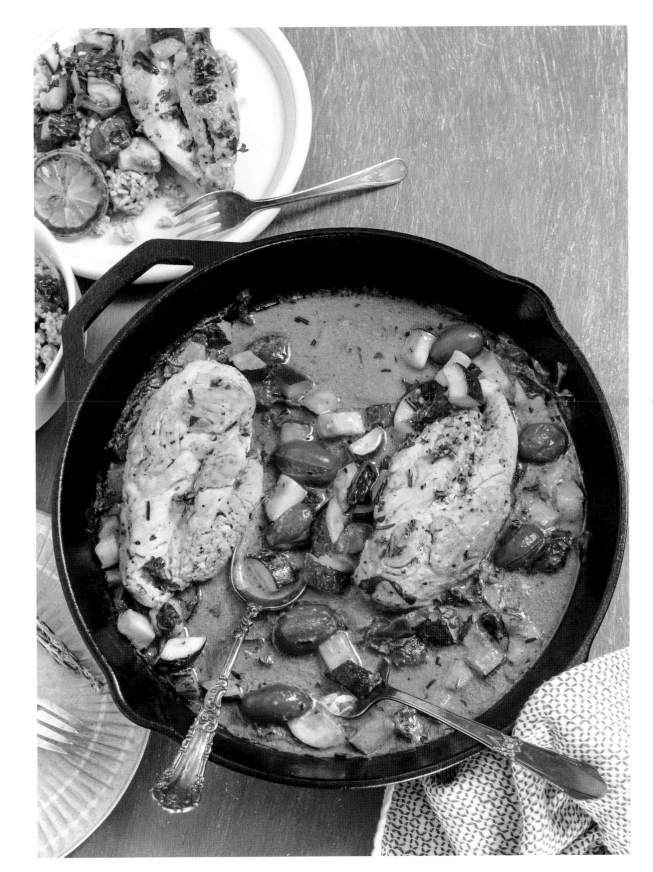

mediterranean red pepper risotto with shrimp

YIELD: 2 servings
PREP TIME: 10 minutes (not including time to cook rice)
COOK TIME: 10 minutes

Funny story: My mom isn't a fan of shrimp or green olives. So naturally, I made this dish for her to see if I could change her mind. She can be stubborn at times! She took one bite—to my surprise, she started with the shrimp and an olive on the fork—and the next thing I knew, she had eaten the entire plate. This meal comes off as elegant and fancy, yet it's ready in about twenty minutes. It is filling but won't leave you feeling overly heavy. Swap the shrimp for the same amount of any white fish, or use portobello mushrooms or cubed tofu in place of the shrimp.

2 tablespoons extra-virgin olive oil

1 pound medium or large shrimp, peeled and deveined

¼ teaspoon coarse sea salt

¼ teaspoon ground black pepper

½ teaspoon ground dried rosemary

¼ cup dry white wine

⅓ cup chopped roasted red peppers, jarred or homemade (see page 96)

3 tablespoons sliced green olives

1 tablespoon fresh squeezed lemon juice

1 cup cooked RightRice (Vegetable Risotto, Wild Mushroom, or Cracked Pepper flavor) or other type of veggie rice, for serving

1. Heat the oil in a large skillet or sauté pan over medium-high heat. Add the shrimp, season with the salt, black pepper, and rosemary, and cook for 3 minutes. Turn the shrimp over and pour in the wine. Simmer until the shrimp turn pink, about 5 minutes.

2. Stir in the roasted red peppers, olives, and lemon juice and remove from the heat.

3. Divide the rice between two plates; top each with half of the shrimp mixture.

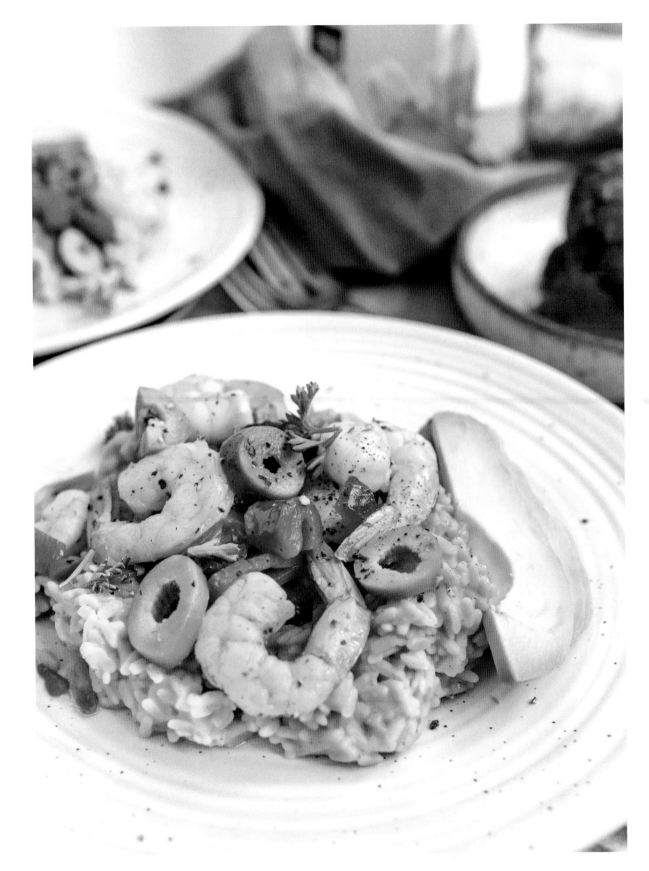

mushroom & brussels sprouts

pizza

YIELD: 1 large pizza (4 servings)

PREP TIME: 15 minutes, plus 4 hours 15 minutes for dough to rest and rise

COOK TIME: 18 minutes

Pizza is a weekly staple in my household—I make a homemade pie most weekends. The secret to achieving the ideal fluffy but crispy crust texture is to use half 00 flour and half all-purpose flour. This filling pizza is loaded with veggies and uses garlic sauce in place of tomato sauce—perfect for a date night in.

CRUST:

1 cup plus 1 tablespoon 00 flour

1 cup plus 1 tablespoon all-purpose flour

1 teaspoon coarse sea salt

¾ teaspoon active dry yeast

¼ teaspoon granulated sugar

1 teaspoon extra-virgin olive oil

1 cup plus 1 tablespoon lukewarm water, divided

TOPPINGS:

6 tablespoons Magic Garlic Sauce (page 216)

½ cup shredded mozzarella or vegan cheese

1 cup thinly sliced baby bella or button mushrooms

1 cup thinly sliced Brussels sprouts

¼ cup sliced red onions

1 teaspoon dried oregano leaves

1 teaspoon sliced fresh basil

Plant-Based Parmesan (page 212), for garnish

Red pepper flakes, for garnish

1. Make the crust: In a large bowl, mix together the flours and salt. In a smaller bowl, whisk the yeast, sugar, oil, and 1 cup of the water until well combined. Add the wet mixture to the flour mixture. Mix together for about 3 minutes. The dough will be very sticky. Add the remaining 1 tablespoon of water and use your hands to knead the dough for another 2 minutes. Let rest for 15 minutes.

2. Turn the dough onto a floured work surface and knead until smooth, then form into a ball. Dust the dough with flour, place in a clean bowl, and cover the bowl with a damp kitchen towel. Let the dough rise at room temperature until it has nearly doubled, 3 to 4 hours.

3. Preheat the oven to 450°F. If using a pizza stone, place it in the oven while the oven preheats.

4. On a floured surface, gently roll the dough into a large, thin circle. Transfer to the preheated pizza stone or a cookie sheet lined with parchment paper.

5. Spread the garlic sauce over the dough. Scatter the cheese over the sauce. Layer the mushrooms, Brussels sprouts, and onions over the cheese. Top with the oregano and basil. Bake for about 18 minutes, until the crust is well browned and the cheese is bubbling; keep a close eye on it toward the end. Remove from the oven and garnish with plant-based parmesan and red pepper flakes. Slice and serve immediately.

meal prep tip: ————————————————

You can make the dough ahead and store it in a sealed container in the fridge for up to 24 hours. It will rise a bit! Bring it to room temperature about 1 hour before baking the pizza.

sunday
burgers

YIELD: 4 burgers
PREP TIME: 5 minutes
COOK TIME: 10 minutes

Every so often, I crave a meat-based meal. These moderately sized burgers will satisfy and are perfect for date night. This recipe was adapted from a Julia Child recipe that my mom found in the newspaper when I was a kid. I've been grilling up these burgers on Sunday nights ever since, making a few changes to give the recipe my own twist, such as adding thyme. The burgers are so savory and full of herby flavor, especially if you use fresh thyme rather than dried. Top them however you like. The sweet potato fries on page 162 make a nice side.

1 pound lean ground beef

⅓ cup finely chopped red onions

2 tablespoons Worcestershire sauce

½ teaspoon fresh thyme leaves, or ¼ teaspoon dried thyme leaves

¼ teaspoon coarse sea salt

¼ teaspoon ground black pepper

¼ to ½ cup crumbled goat cheese, or 4 slices cheese of choice (optional)

1 large tomato, sliced

1 small head romaine lettuce, leaves separated, or 4 burger buns

Burger toppings of choice

1. Preheat a grill to medium-high heat.

2. Put the ground beef, red onions, Worcestershire sauce, thyme, salt, and pepper in a medium glass or ceramic mixing bowl and mix well with your hands. Form into four equal-sized patties, 1½ to 2 inches thick.

3. Once the grill is hot, grill the patties for 4 to 5 minutes before flipping. Grill the other side for 3 minutes for medium or 4 to 5 minutes for well-done burgers. Top with the cheese, if using, and close the lid for 1 minute to melt it.

4. Top the burgers with tomato slices and the other toppings of your choice and serve wrapped in romaine lettuce leaves or on traditional burger buns.

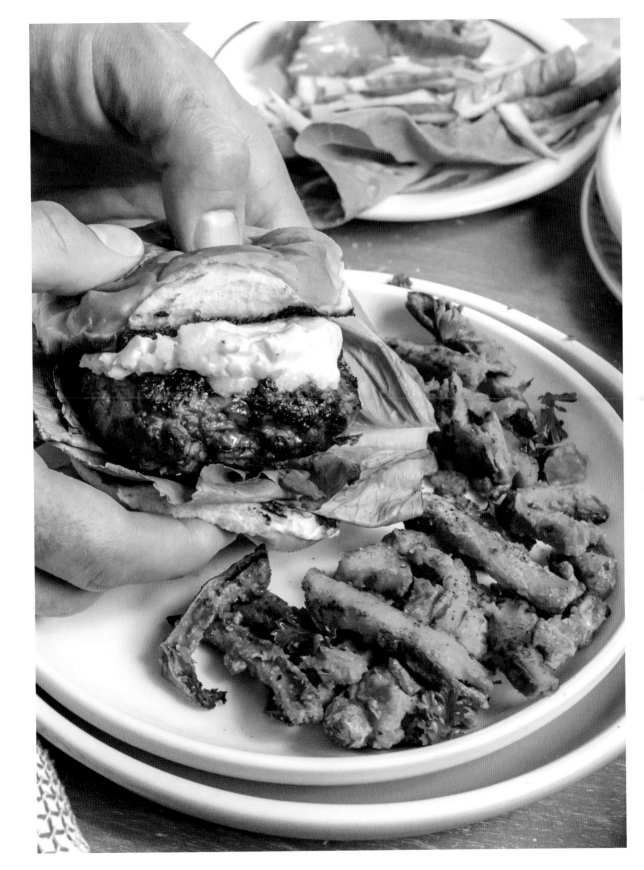

sweet potato
tacos

YIELD: <u>8 to 10 tacos (2 per serving)</u>
PREP TIME: <u>20 minutes (not including time to make sauce or walnut meat)</u>
COOK TIME: <u>20 minutes</u>

Be prepared to blow your partner's socks off with these tacos. I make them spicy, but you can omit the cayenne pepper or swap in paprika to make them milder. They have a smoky bite, and the walnut meat gives them a nice texture while the garlic cream sauce cuts the heat and leaves you craving more. This dish was a favorite in my family while I was testing new recipes for this cookbook, and I have made it several times since!

1 large sweet potato

1 teaspoon chipotle powder

½ teaspoon coarse sea salt

¼ teaspoon cayenne pepper

1 tablespoon extra-virgin olive oil

WALNUT MEAT:

1 cup raw walnuts

1 tablespoon coconut aminos or soy sauce

½ teaspoon garlic powder

½ teaspoon ground dried oregano

¼ teaspoon coarse sea salt

8 to 10 small white corn or flour tortillas

1 cup Magic Garlic Sauce (page 216)

1 cup arugula

FOR GARNISH (OPTIONAL):

Avocado slices

Red onion slices

Fresh cilantro leaves

1. Preheat the oven to 375°F. Line a rimmed baking sheet with parchment paper.

2. Peel and dice the sweet potato. Place in a bowl and toss with the chipotle powder, salt, and cayenne, followed by the oil. Be sure all the potato pieces are well coated on all sides.

3. Spread the seasoned sweet potato in a single layer on the prepared baking sheet. Bake for 20 minutes, or until the potatoes are soft and can easily be pierced with a fork. Remove from the oven and let cool a bit.

4. Meanwhile, make the walnut meat: Place all the ingredients in a food processor or high-powered blender and pulse until well combined and crumbly.

5. If desired, char the tortillas over an open flame on the stovetop.

6. Fill the tortillas with a drizzle of garlic sauce, the arugula, sweet potatoes, and 1 to 2 tablespoons of walnut meat. Garnish as desired and enjoy!

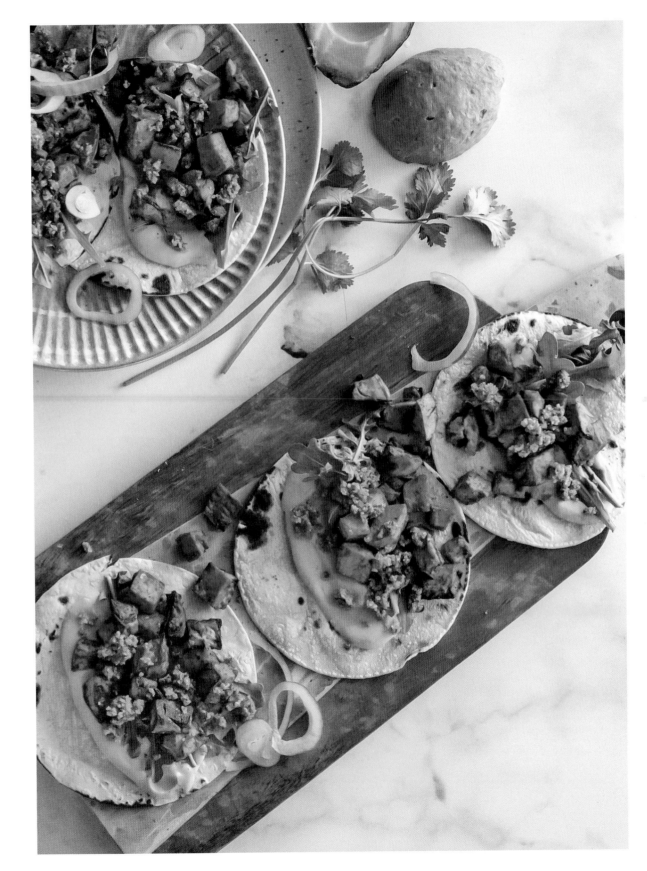

plant-based tuscan alfredo
with artichokes & mushrooms

YIELD: <u>4 servings</u>
PREP TIME: <u>10 minutes (not including time to make Plant-Based Parmesan)</u>
COOK TIME: <u>20 minutes</u>

Pasta is the best food for date night, in my humble opinion. I recommend making this recipe with your partner mainly because it calls for white wine, which means you get to finish the bottle with dinner (so pick something you like to drink!). If you don't want to finish a bottle, grab a single-serving bottle of chardonnay for this recipe. You will be eating loads of garlic, so neither of you will notice the garlic breath. Add chicken or shrimp for more protein.

This recipe makes quite a bit of leftovers, at least in my house. Leftovers will keep in an airtight container in the refrigerator for up to 4 days.

8 ounces fettuccine

3 tablespoons extra-virgin olive oil

5 cloves garlic, chopped (about 2 tablespoons)

1 (12-ounce) can quartered artichoke hearts, drained

1¼ cups grape or cherry tomatoes

1 cup sliced mushrooms

3½ teaspoons arrowroot starch or cornstarch

2 cups So Delicious Original coconut milk creamer or SILK unsweetened almond milk, divided, plus more if needed

¼ cup dry white wine

½ teaspoon coarse sea salt

½ teaspoon ground black pepper

½ teaspoon garlic powder

½ teaspoon onion powder

¼ cup plus 2 tablespoons nutritional yeast

3 tablespoons Plant-Based Parmesan (page 212)

Chopped fresh parsley, for garnish

1. Cook the fettuccine in a pot of salted water according to the package directions. Once you add the pasta to the boiling water, start the sauce.

2. Heat the oil in a large skillet or sauté pan over medium heat. Reduce the heat to medium-low and add the garlic, artichoke hearts, tomatoes, and mushrooms. Cook until the mushrooms start to soften a little, about 5 minutes.

3. Meanwhile, make a slurry by mixing the arrowroot with 1 cup of the creamer, stirring until there are no lumps.

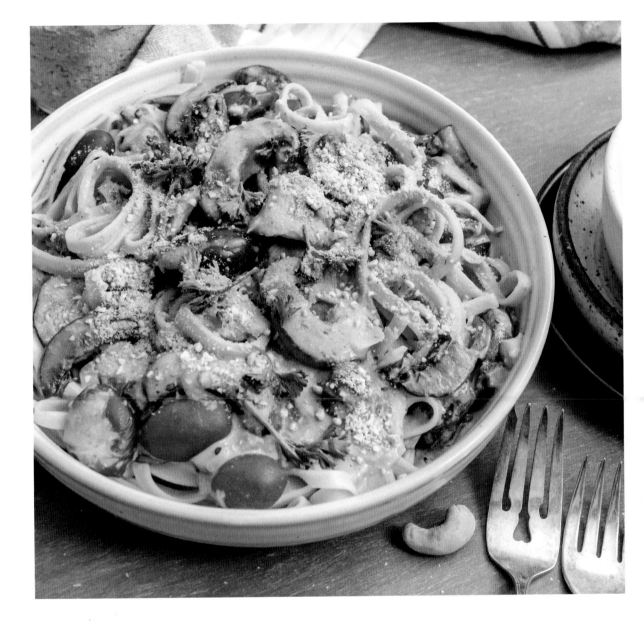

4. Pour the remaining 1 cup of creamer and the wine over the veggies in the skillet and bring to a simmer. Stir in the salt, pepper, garlic powder, onion powder, and slurry. Turn the heat down to low and simmer until the sauce has thickened, about 5 more minutes. Feel free to add ½ cup more creamer at a time if the sauce seems too thick.

5. Drain the fettuccine, pour the sauce over the pasta, and mix well. Top each serving with the plant-based parmesan, garnish with parsley, and enjoy.

teriyaki salmon
sheet pan dinner

YIELD: 2 servings
PREP TIME: 10 minutes, plus
10 minutes to marinate salmon
COOK TIME: 20 minutes

This is an easy, fresh dinner for you and a plus-one to share. You won't have many dishes to clean since everything cooks nicely on one pan in the oven. The teriyaki sauce really complements the salmon, but feel free to substitute boneless, skinless chicken breast or portobello mushroom caps.

⅓ cup teriyaki sauce, homemade (page 211) or store-bought

1 (½-inch) piece fresh ginger, peeled and chopped

1½ teaspoons red pepper flakes

½ teaspoon garlic powder

1 (1-pound) skin-on salmon fillet

8 ounces Brussels sprouts, thinly sliced lengthwise

1 cup cooked RightRice or other type of veggie rice, for serving

2 tablespoons chopped green onions, for garnish

1. In a large bowl, whisk together the teriyaki sauce, ginger, red pepper flakes, and garlic powder. Add the salmon and allow to marinate for about 10 minutes.

2. Preheat the oven to 375°F. Line a rimmed baking sheet with parchment paper.

3. Remove the salmon from the marinade (reserve the marinade) and place the fish skin side down on one half of the prepared pan. Arrange the Brussels sprouts in a single layer on the other half of the pan. Pour the reserved marinade over the salmon and vegetables.

4. Bake until the salmon is cooked to your desired doneness, 18 to 20 minutes for well-done.

5. Divide the rice between two plates, top with the salmon, and place the Brussels sprouts on the side. Garnish with the green onions.

tip:

If you're not up for making homemade teriyaki sauce, I like Trader Joe's Soyaki Sauce for this recipe.

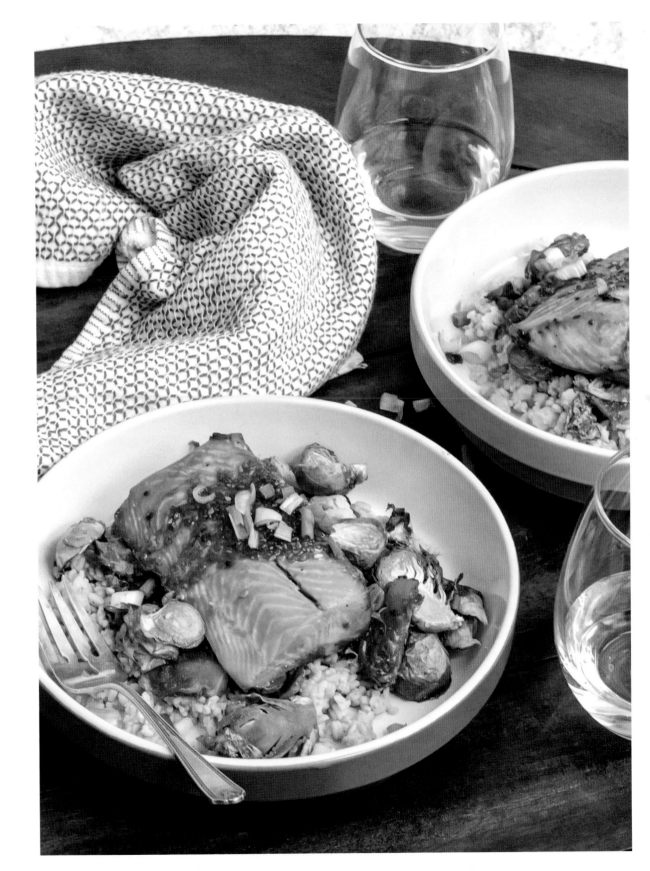

chapter 5

salads & sides

Baked Spiced Cauliflower | 151

Superfood Salad with
Lemon Honey Dressing | 152

Harvest Salad with Maple Vinaigrette | 154

Fiesta Salad with Plant-Based Ranch | 156

Roasted Veggie Salad | 158

Shrimp Cobb Salad | 160

Sweet Potato Fries with Parmesan | 162

Parsnip Fries | 164

Peanut Butter Brussels Sprouts | 166

baked spiced
cauliflower

YIELD: 2 to 4 servings
PREP TIME: 10 minutes
COOK TIME: 30 minutes

This cauliflower is delicious. You can eat it on its own or serve it as a side dish with any of the dinners in this book. You could also serve it as an appetizer with Plant-Based Ranch Dressing (page 156), Red Pepper Sauce (page 116), or Romesco Dip (page 180).

1 tablespoon garlic powder

1½ teaspoons onion powder

1 teaspoon chili powder

½ teaspoon paprika

½ teaspoon ground black pepper

½ teaspoon coarse sea salt

5 to 6 cups chopped cauliflower (from about 1 medium to large head)

2 tablespoons extra-virgin olive oil

Chopped fresh parsley, for garnish

1. Preheat the oven to 400°F. Line a rimmed baking sheet with parchment paper.

2. In a small bowl, whisk together the spices and salt. Put the cauliflower in a large bowl, sprinkle the spice mixture over the cauliflower, and toss well. Pour the oil over the spiced cauliflower and toss again to coat.

3. Spread the cauliflower in a single layer on the prepared baking sheet. Bake until browned and soft, about 30 minutes. Serve garnished with parsley.

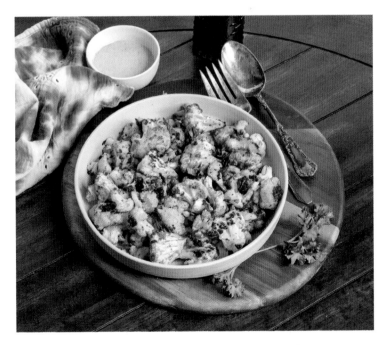

superfood salad
with lemon honey dressing

YIELD: 4 servings
PREP TIME: 15 minutes (not including time to cook quinoa)

This salad is one of my most popular recipes to date. The creamy dairy-free dressing full of feel-good ingredients is the true star of this recipe, so be sure not to skimp on that! It's a very filling salad with lots of great texture from the massaged kale and quinoa.

6 cups stemmed and chopped kale

1 tablespoon extra-virgin olive oil

1 cup cooked quinoa

1 cup diced cucumbers

½ cup chopped tomatoes

2 cups baby spinach (optional)

1 avocado, sliced

LEMON HONEY DRESSING:

¼ cup tahini, stirred well

¼ cup warm water

1 tablespoon plus 1 teaspoon fresh squeezed lemon juice

1 teaspoon honey

¼ teaspoon minced garlic

⅛ teaspoon coarse sea salt

1. In a large bowl, combine the kale and olive oil. Gently massage the kale with your hands to soften the leaves. Add the quinoa, cucumbers, tomatoes, and spinach, if using. Mix well.

2. Make the dressing: Put the tahini in a small bowl. Slowly add the warm water and mix with a whisk or fork. Keep mixing in small amounts of water until the tahini "accepts" the water. It takes a little patience and trust, but it will eventually thin to a dressing consistency. Once it reaches your preferred consistency, add the lemon juice, honey, garlic, and salt and whisk well.

3. Pour the dressing over the salad and toss well before serving.

meal prep tip:

This salad holds up well in the fridge, so it's a good choice for meal prep. It tastes even better a day or two later.

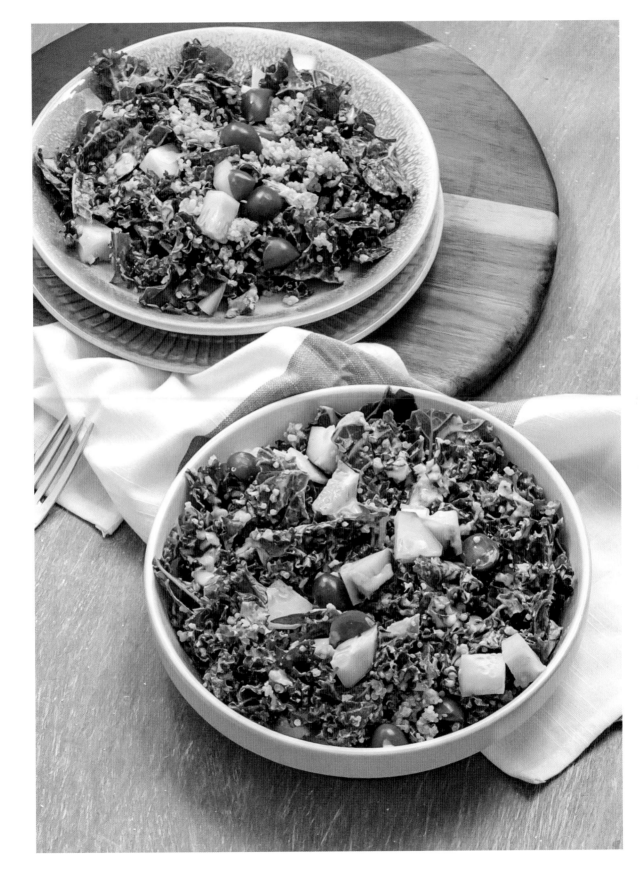

harvest salad
with maple vinaigrette

YIELD: 4 servings

PREP TIME: 8 minutes (not including time to cook quinoa)

COOK TIME: 20 minutes

You will love the flavors of this crowd-pleaser of a salad. It is perfect for the fall season, but since the ingredients are easy to find, it can be made any time of the year. The salad is completely plant-based; however, you can top it with cooked chicken, salmon, or shrimp to make it a bit more filling. The dressing is full of fall flavors, with sweet notes from the maple and a nice tang from the vinegar.

1 medium sweet potato, peeled and chopped

1 medium acorn squash, peeled and chopped

1 cup halved Brussels sprouts

2 tablespoons extra-virgin olive oil

1 tablespoon garlic powder

1½ teaspoons onion powder

1½ teaspoons paprika

½ teaspoon coarse sea salt

1 (5- to 6-ounce) package baby spinach

2 cups stemmed and finely chopped kale

1 cup cooked quinoa

1 cup diced or sliced apples (any variety)

MAPLE VINAIGRETTE:

⅓ cup extra-virgin olive oil

3 tablespoons water

1½ tablespoons apple cider vinegar

1½ tablespoons maple syrup

½ teaspoon coarse sea salt

½ teaspoon minced onions

¼ teaspoon paprika

1. Preheat the oven to 375°F. Line a rimmed baking sheet with parchment paper.

2. Put the sweet potato, acorn squash, and Brussels sprouts in a large bowl. Add the oil, garlic powder, onion powder, paprika, and salt and toss well to fully coat the veggies. Spread the veggies in a single layer on the prepared baking sheet and roast until fork-tender, about 20 minutes.

3. Meanwhile, make the vinaigrette: Put all the ingredients in a medium bowl. If you have an immersion blender, use it to emulsify the dressing until it is thick and creamy. If not, whisk the ingredients well by hand or place them in a jar with a tight-fitting lid and shake to combine. If the dressing is too thick, add another 1 tablespoon of water.

4. Arrange the spinach and kale in a large serving bowl, top with the quinoa and roasted veggies, and toss well. Pour in the dressing, then add the apples. Toss again to be sure all the greens are evenly coated with the dressing. You may also plate the salad and drizzle the dressing over the top.

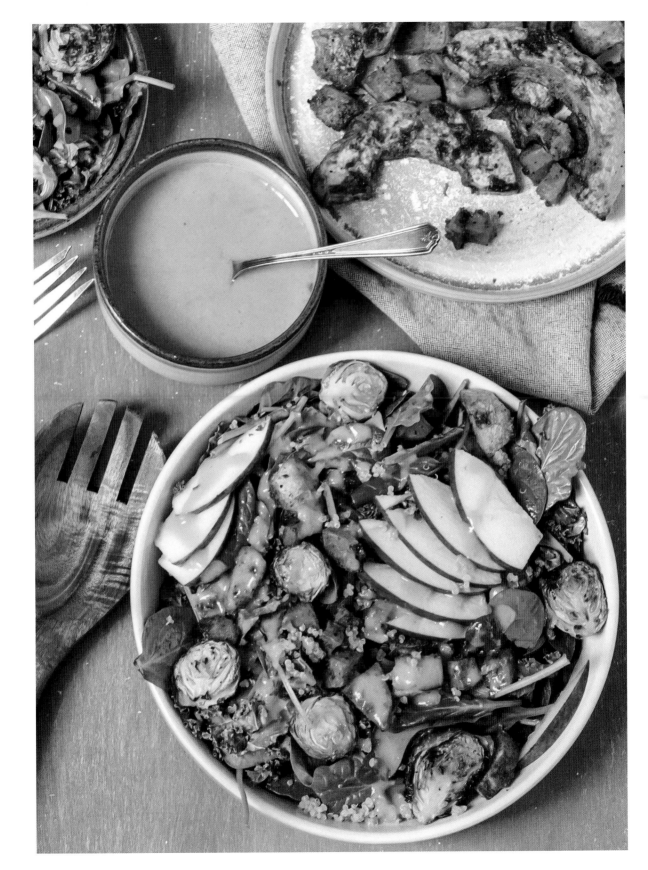

fiesta salad
with plant-based ranch

YIELD: 4 servings
PREP TIME: 10 minutes
COOK TIME: 12 minutes

This salad is a party in your mouth. Mixing Mexican-inspired flavors with a plant-based ranch dressing creates a savory concoction that you will crave.

1 tablespoon extra-virgin olive oil

1 cup frozen corn kernels

1 cup chopped zucchini

¼ cup chopped onions

1 cup canned black beans, drained and rinsed

½ teaspoon chili powder

½ teaspoon paprika

¼ teaspoon coarse sea salt

¼ teaspoon ground black pepper

1 (10- to 11-ounce) package mixed greens or baby spinach

PLANT-BASED RANCH DRESSING:

⅓ cup tahini, stirred well

⅓ cup warm water

3 tablespoons fresh squeezed lemon juice

1 tablespoon chopped fresh dill

1 tablespoon Dijon mustard

1½ teaspoons white miso

1 clove garlic, minced

½ teaspoon honey

¼ teaspoon onion powder

FOR GARNISH/SERVING (OPTIONAL):

Avocado slices

Chopped roasted red peppers

Black and/or white sesame seeds

Chopped fresh cilantro

Lime wedges

1. Heat the oil in a large skillet over high heat. Add the corn, zucchini, onions, black beans, chili powder, paprika, salt, and pepper and stir well to make sure all the veggies are coated. Sauté until the veggies are softened and the zucchini is starting to brown, 8 to 12 minutes. Take the pan off the heat and set the veggie mixture aside.

2. Make the dressing: If using an immersion blender, put all the ingredients in a medium bowl and blend until smooth. If whisking by hand, put the tahini and warm water in a medium bowl and whisk well, then add the remaining dressing ingredients and whisk to combine. You may need to add another tablespoon or two of water to achieve the desired consistency.

3. Layer the greens in 4 serving bowls, top with the veggie mixture, and garnish with avocado slices, roasted red peppers, sesame seeds, and/or cilantro, if desired. Drizzle the dressing over the salads. Serve with lime wedges, if desired.

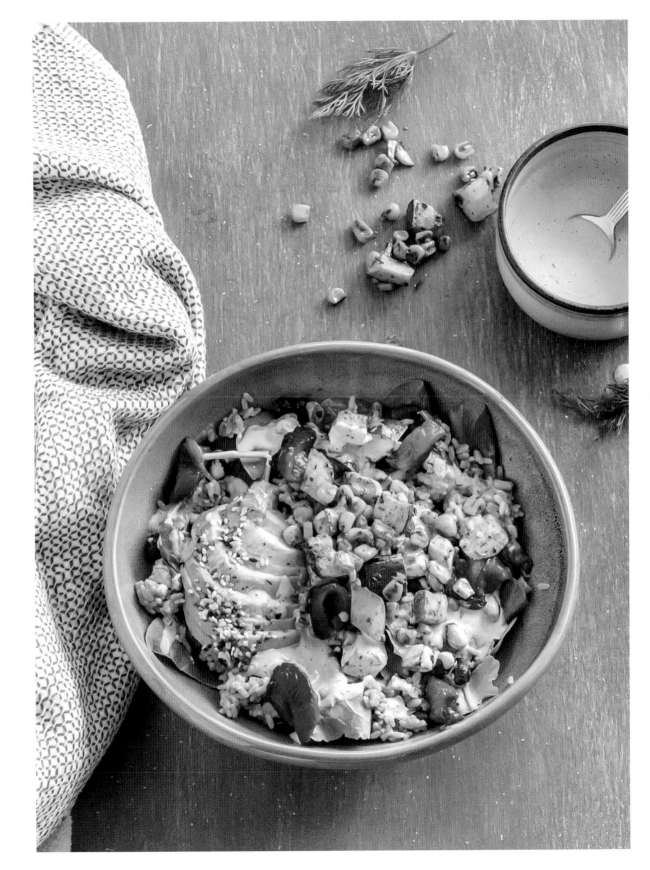

roasted veggie
salad

YIELD: 4 servings

PREP TIME: 15 minutes (not including time to cook rice or make dressing)

COOK TIME: 30 minutes

This salad is satisfying without being loaded with calories. You can use any veggies you prefer, but I find that sweet potato and cauliflower pair especially well with these particular seasonings. You can also use any dressing you like, but I recommend my Magic Garlic Dressing. Buy preroasted garlic cloves to cut down on prep time!

2 cups peeled and chopped sweet potatoes (about 2 medium)

2 cups chopped cauliflower (about 1 small head)

1 cup chopped broccoli

1 tablespoon curry powder

1 tablespoon garlic powder

1 tablespoon onion powder

1 tablespoon paprika

½ teaspoon coarse sea salt

1 teaspoon red pepper flakes

2 tablespoons extra-virgin olive oil

1 (10- to 11-ounce) package mixed greens or baby spinach

1 cup cooked wild rice blend, cooled

½ cup Magic Garlic Dressing (page 216)

1 avocado, sliced, for garnish (optional)

1. Preheat the oven to 400°F and line a rimmed baking sheet with parchment paper.

2. Put the sweet potatoes, cauliflower, and broccoli in a large bowl. In a small bowl, whisk together the curry powder, garlic powder, onion powder, paprika, salt, and red pepper flakes. Pour the seasoning mixture over the vegetables and toss well. Drizzle with the oil and toss again, making sure all the vegetables are thoroughly coated.

3. Spread the seasoned vegetables in a single layer on the prepared baking sheet. Roast until they are cooked through and can easily be pieced with a fork, about 30 minutes. Set aside.

4. Divide the greens among four plates and toss each portion with ¼ cup of the wild rice. Arrange the roasted veggies on top and drizzle with the dressing. Garnish with avocado slices, if desired.

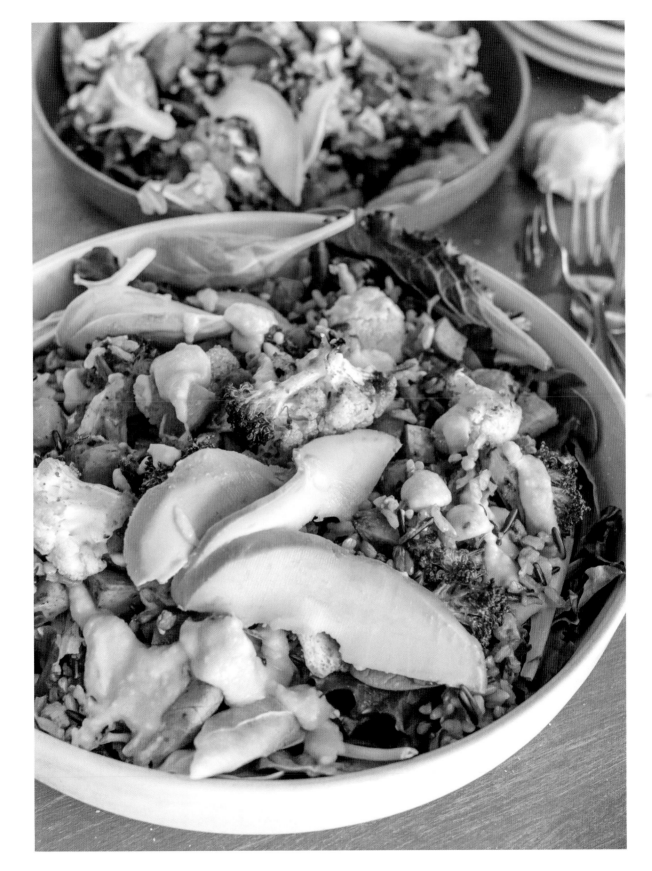

shrimp cobb
salad

YIELD: 2 servings
PREP TIME: 10 minutes (not including time to hard-boil eggs)
COOK TIME: 8 minutes

This salad is packed with protein and flavor. It is dairy-free; you won't miss the blue cheese or the buttermilk in the quick and easy ranch dressing, and you won't feel heavy after your meal. Although shrimp is my favorite protein topper for this salad, I have also made it with grilled chicken, with salmon, and even with no meat at all.

SHRIMP:

6 ounces medium shrimp

½ teaspoon ranch seasoning

¼ teaspoon coarse sea salt

¼ teaspoon ground black pepper

1 tablespoon extra-virgin olive oil

EASY RANCH DRESSING:

¼ cup plus 1 tablespoon tahini, stirred well

1½ tablespoons ranch seasoning

¼ cup warm water

¼ cup fresh squeezed lemon juice

1 teaspoon Dijon mustard

SALAD:

6 cups chopped romaine lettuce

4 hard-boiled eggs, peeled

1 Hass avocado, peeled, pitted, and sliced

¼ cup halved grape tomatoes

2 tablespoons thinly sliced red onions

1. Peel, devein, and tail the shrimp. Rub the shrimp with the ranch seasoning, salt, and pepper. Heat the oil in a medium skillet over medium-high heat. When hot, add the shrimp and cook for 4 minutes on each side, or until they are light pink in color and opaque throughout. Set aside.

2. Meanwhile, make the dressing: In a bowl, whisk together the tahini and ranch seasoning. Add the warm water 2 tablespoons at a time, whisking after each addition. Continue to mix until the dressing is pourable. Add the lemon juice and mustard and mix well. Set aside.

3. Assemble the salad: Put the lettuce in a large bowl. Chop or slice the hard-boiled eggs. Arrange the eggs, avocado slices, tomatoes, and onions on top of the lettuce; toss well, if desired. Drizzle with the dressing and top with the shrimp.

tip:

Yes, you can make a ranch-style seasoning mix from scratch, but to me, it just doesn't taste as "ranchy." I like Simply Organic brand ranch seasoning.

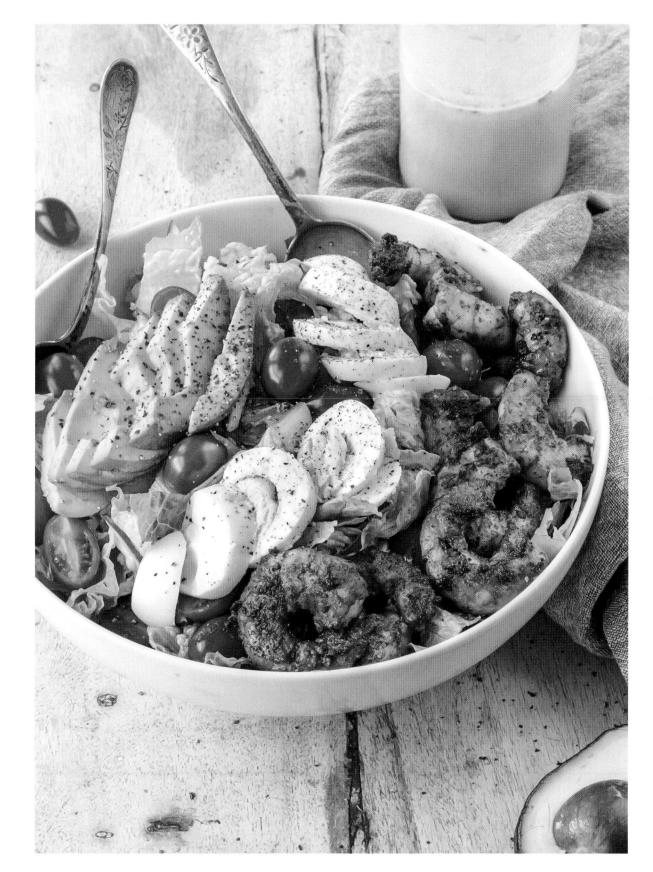

sweet potato fries
with parmesan

YIELD: 2 to 4 servings
PREP TIME: 10 minutes
COOK TIME: 25 minutes

Sweet potato fries are my kryptonite. I could eat two potatoes' worth of fries a day with any meal, but I try not to. I play around with so many different fry flavors, and this recipe is my current favorite.

2 medium sweet potatoes, cut into even fry shapes

½ teaspoon garlic powder

½ teaspoon kosher salt

¼ teaspoon ground black pepper

¼ teaspoon onion powder

1 tablespoon extra-virgin olive oil

⅓ cup grated Parmesan or Pecorino Romano cheese

Artichoke Pesto (page 72) or Plant-Based Ranch Dressing (page 156), for serving

1. Preheat the oven to 400°F. Line a rimmed baking sheet with parchment paper.

2. In a large bowl, toss the sweet potato fries with the garlic powder, salt, pepper, and onion powder. Add the oil and toss again to ensure that the fries are evenly coated.

3. Spread the fries in a single layer on the prepared baking sheet, being mindful not to overlap them. Bake until crispy, 20 to 25 minutes, tossing the fries halfway through baking.

4. Return the fries to the bowl, sprinkle the cheese over them, and toss well. Serve with pesto or ranch.

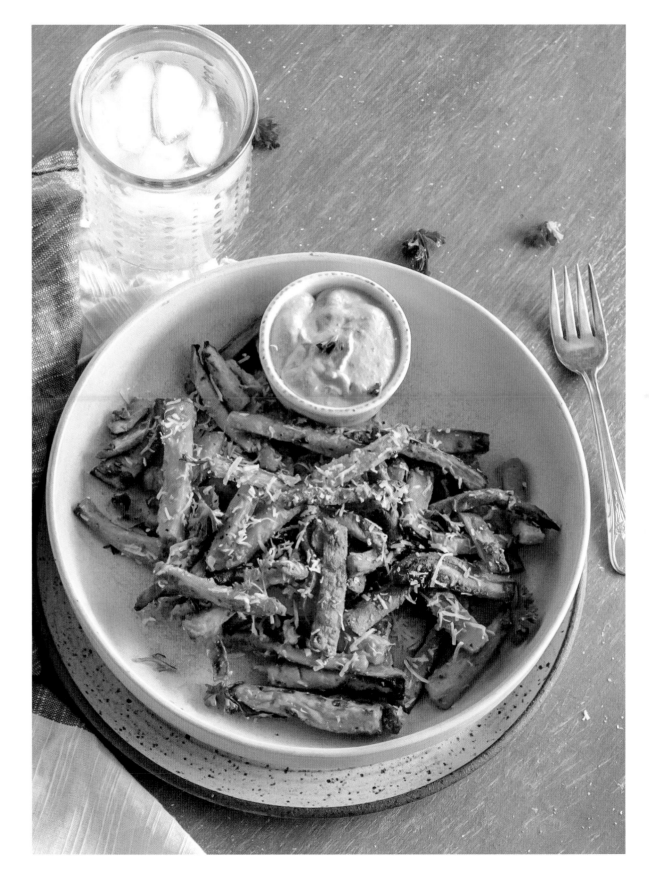

parsnip
fries

YIELD: <u>4 servings</u>
PREP TIME: <u>10 minutes</u>
COOK TIME: <u>25 minutes</u>

When I need a fun change from my go-to sweet potato fries (page 162), I opt for parsnip fries. You may find that you don't even need a dipping sauce. Pair them with Sneaky Turkey Meatloaf (page 110) or Sunday Burgers (page 142) or use them to top any salad.

1 pound parsnips

1 tablespoon grated Parmesan cheese

½ teaspoon coarse sea salt

½ teaspoon chipotle powder

½ teaspoon garlic powder

½ teaspoon paprika

¼ teaspoon onion powder

1 tablespoon extra-virgin olive oil

½ teaspoon chopped fresh parsley, for garnish (optional)

1. Preheat the oven to 375°F. Line a rimmed baking sheet with parchment paper.

2. Peel the parsnips and slice into fry shapes; try to make them similar in size so they cook evenly. (This step can be a little tricky given the typical irregular shape of a parsnip.)

3. In a small bowl, mix together the Parmesan cheese, salt, and spices. Put the parsnip fries in a large bowl, sprinkle the seasoning mixture over them, and toss well to ensure all the fries are coated. Drizzle the oil over the seasoned fries and toss again to ensure that the fries are evenly coated.

4. Spread the fries in a single layer on the prepared baking sheet, being mindful not to overlap them. Bake for 20 minutes, toss well, and bake for another 5 minutes, or until crispy. Garnish with parsley, if desired.

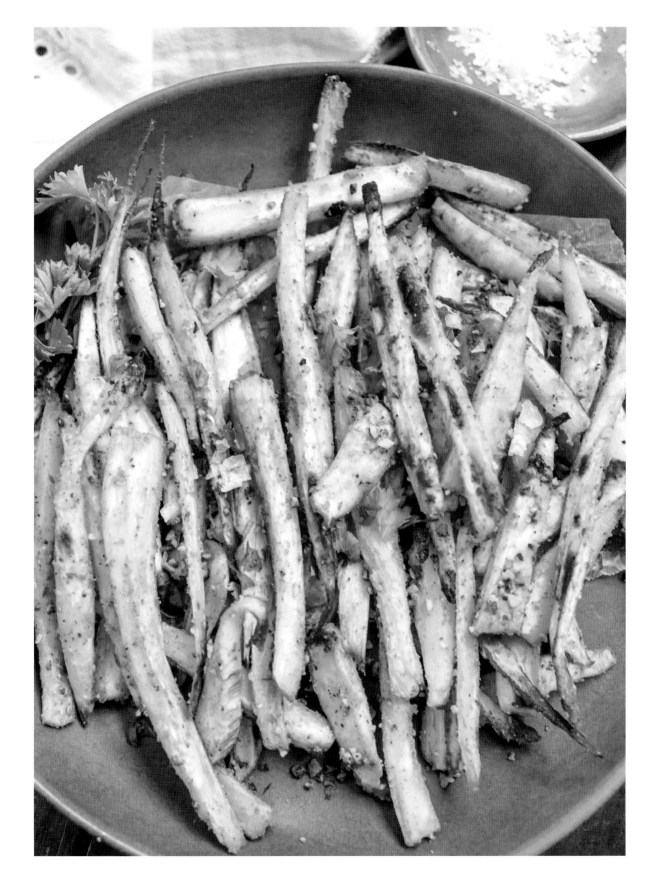

peanut butter
brussels sprouts

YIELD: 4 servings
PREP TIME: 10 minutes
COOK TIME: 30 minutes

These Brussels sprouts are creamy, sweet, savory, and highly addictive. They make the perfect side dish for all sorts of meals. They are filling and give off a Thai-inspired flavor you don't typically expect from a veggie.

2 pounds Brussels sprouts

2 tablespoons extra-virgin olive oil

1½ teaspoons garlic powder

¼ teaspoon coarse sea salt

⅛ teaspoon ground black pepper

¼ cup natural creamy peanut butter

1½ teaspoons soy sauce

¼ cup water, or more if needed to thin the sauce

⅓ cup dried cranberries

⅓ cup raw pecans

1. Preheat the oven to 400°F. Line a rimmed baking sheet with parchment paper.

2. Slice the Brussels sprouts into halves or quarters depending on how large they are and place them in a large bowl. Sprinkle with the oil, garlic powder, salt, and pepper and toss to coat.

3. Spread the sprouts on the prepared baking sheet and bake for 30 minutes, tossing regularly to ensure they cook evenly.

4. Meanwhile, whisk together the peanut butter, soy sauce, and water. If the sauce is too thick to spread evenly, add another tablespoon or two of water. Taste the sauce and add a pinch of salt if needed.

5. Add the cranberries, pecans, and peanut butter sauce to the Brussels sprouts and mix well to coat the sprouts with the sauce and evenly distribute the berries and nuts. If desired, pop the pan back in the oven for another 3 to 5 minutes to warm everything up a bit, or serve immediately.

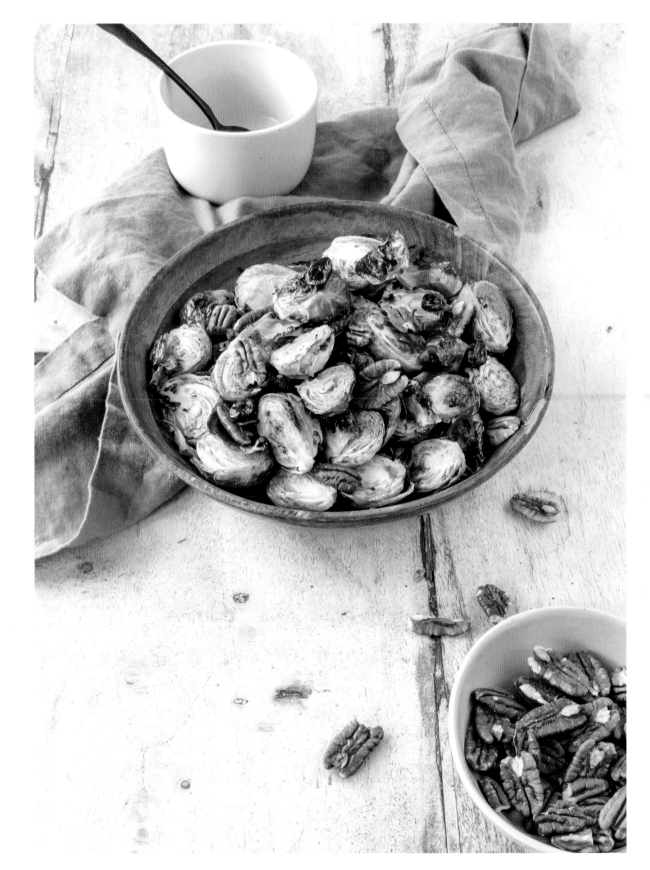

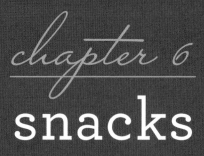

chapter 6

snacks

Strawberry Bliss Balls | 169

Blueberry Banana Bread | 170

No-Bake Trail Mix Bars | 172

Oatmeal Funfetti Mug Cake | 174

Pumpkin Zucchini Bread | 176

Hummus | 178

Romesco Dip | 180

Savory Nuts | 182

Quinoa-Stuffed Mushrooms | 184

Savory Herbaceous Popcorn | 186

Sweet Graham Cracker Popcorn | 187

strawberry bliss
balls

YIELD: about 10 balls (5 servings)
PREP TIME: 10 minutes

These bliss balls are the perfect healthier treat for when you need something lightly sweet, or you can pop one or two for a pre- or post-workout snack. I like mine flavored with freeze-dried strawberries, which you can find in the nut and dried fruit aisle of most grocery stores. You can use any other freeze-dried fruit to get the flavor you want.

6 pitted dates, soaked in warm water for about 15 minutes and drained

1¼ cups freeze-dried strawberries

1 cup almond butter

½ cup old-fashioned oats

2½ tablespoons melted coconut oil

2 tablespoons maple syrup

2 tablespoons unsweetened coconut flakes, or an additional 1 tablespoon old-fashioned oats

½ teaspoon vanilla or almond extract

Pulse all the ingredients in a food processor until crumbly and slightly sticky. Roll into 1-inch balls with your hands; you should get about 10 balls. Enjoy right away, or store in an airtight container in the refrigerator for up to a week or in the freezer for up to 2 months.

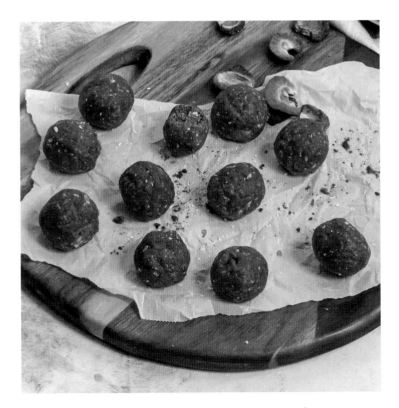

blueberry
banana bread

YIELD: 8 servings
PREP TIME: 8 minutes
COOK TIME: 55 minutes

This bread is based on my mom's banana bread recipe, which has been in my family for quite some time. I will forever think of baking with my mom throughout my childhood when I make this recipe. Over the years, I have, of course, made it my own by making it healthier and adding blueberries and granola to it to create interesting textures and flavors. If you prefer, leave out the granola for a smoother, lighter bread.

1½ cups all-purpose flour

⅔ cup coconut sugar or granulated sugar

1 teaspoon baking powder

½ teaspoon baking soda

½ teaspoon ground cinnamon

½ teaspoon ground nutmeg

3 overripe bananas, mashed

⅓ cup melted coconut oil or butter

2 large eggs, room temperature, lightly beaten

1 teaspoon vanilla extract

1 cup fresh or frozen blueberries

1 cup granola, homemade (page 56) or store-bought (optional)

1. Preheat the oven to 350°F. Grease a 9 by 5-inch or 8½ by 4½-inch loaf pan.

2. In a large bowl, whisk together the flour, sugar, baking powder, baking soda, cinnamon, and nutmeg until no lumps remain. In a separate bowl, whisk together the mashed bananas, coconut oil, eggs, and vanilla until well blended. With a rubber spatula, incorporate the dry mixture into the wet mixture, smoothing out any lumps. Fold in the blueberries and granola, if using.

3. Pour the batter into the prepared pan and bake until a toothpick inserted into the center comes out clean, about 55 minutes. Let cool completely before slicing.

4. Store in an airtight container on the counter for up to 4 days, or freeze for up to 3 months.

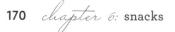

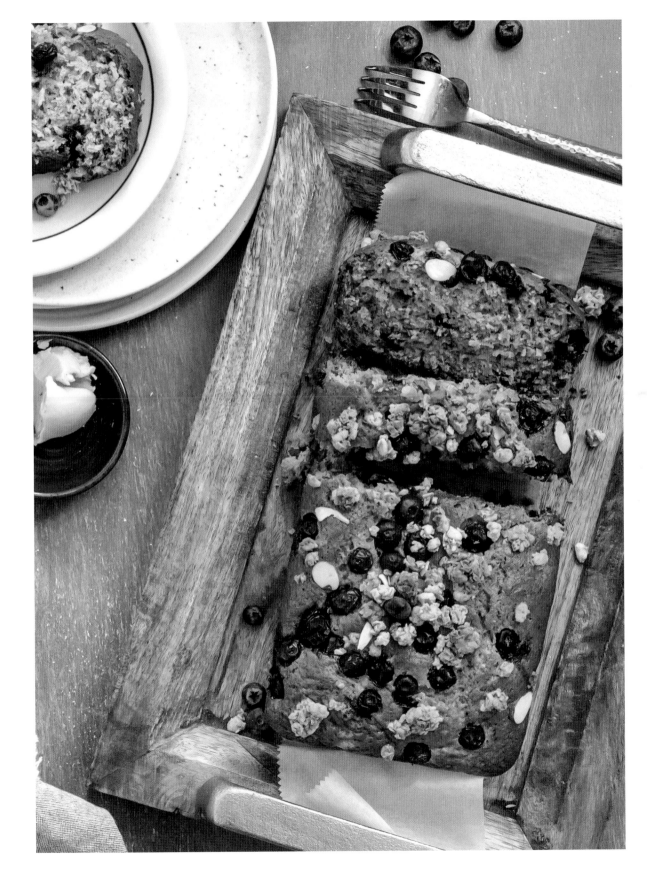

no-bake trail
mix bars

YIELD: 16 bars
PREP TIME: 15 minutes

These bars will be your new favorite sweet treat, I can assure you! They are great for on the go, and they can easily be prepped for the week ahead.

1½ cups old-fashioned oats

1½ cups raw almonds

½ cup dried cranberries

½ cup almond butter

½ cup maple syrup

¼ cup raw walnuts

2 teaspoons vanilla extract

½ teaspoon coarse sea salt

½ cup chocolate chips or roughly chopped chocolate

1. Place all the ingredients except the chocolate in a food processor or high-powered blender. Process for a few minutes until the mixture is thick and crumbly but holds together when you squeeze it with your hand. You may need to remove the lid and loosen the mixture with a rubber spatula a few times. Once the ingredients are well blended, add the chocolate and pulse a couple of times to mix it in while keeping the pieces intact.

2. Line a 9-inch square baking pan with parchment paper. (Or you can use a smaller dish for thicker squares.) Spread the mixture in the pan, pressing down firmly until the top is even.

3. Cut into 16 bars. If the mixture is too sticky to cut, refrigerate it for an hour uncovered and then cut once it is chilled. Store the bars in an airtight container in the refrigerator for up to a week.

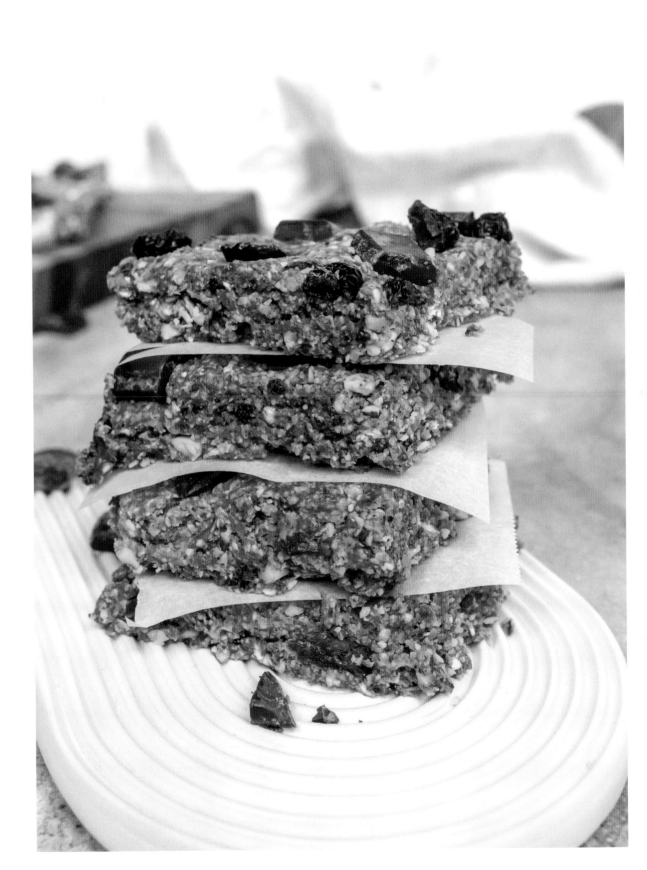

oatmeal funfetti
mug cake

YIELD: 2 servings
PREP TIME: 5 minutes
COOK TIME: 90 seconds

This recipe is almost too easy to be true. Mug cakes started out as an Instagram trend and have since made a weekly appearance in my home for breakfast. This is also a great recipe if you are craving something sweet but healthy and you don't feel like turning on the oven. I made this recipe ten times just for this cookbook—I am not even kidding. As easy as it is, I wanted the cake to have a specific flavor and texture, and perfecting it was a science! This concoction has by far the best flavor and texture. Feel free to use less maple syrup if you are watching your sugar intake.

¾ cup blanched almond flour

¼ cup old-fashioned oats

1 teaspoon baking powder

¼ cup maple syrup

2 tablespoons So Delicious unsweetened coconut milk

1 large egg, lightly beaten

1 teaspoon vanilla extract

2 tablespoons melted coconut oil

2 tablespoons sprinkles (optional)

2 tablespoons So Delicious CocoWhip

In a medium bowl, whisk together the almond flour, oats, and baking powder. Add the maple syrup, milk, egg, and vanilla and mix to combine. Stir in the melted coconut oil and sprinkles, if using. Divide the batter evenly between two medium mugs or ramekins. Microwave on high one at a time for 80 to 90 seconds. Top each cake with a tablespoon of CocoWhip and enjoy.

meal prep tip:

You can make these mug cakes a night or two in advance and keep them chilled; they taste great cold right out of the refrigerator.

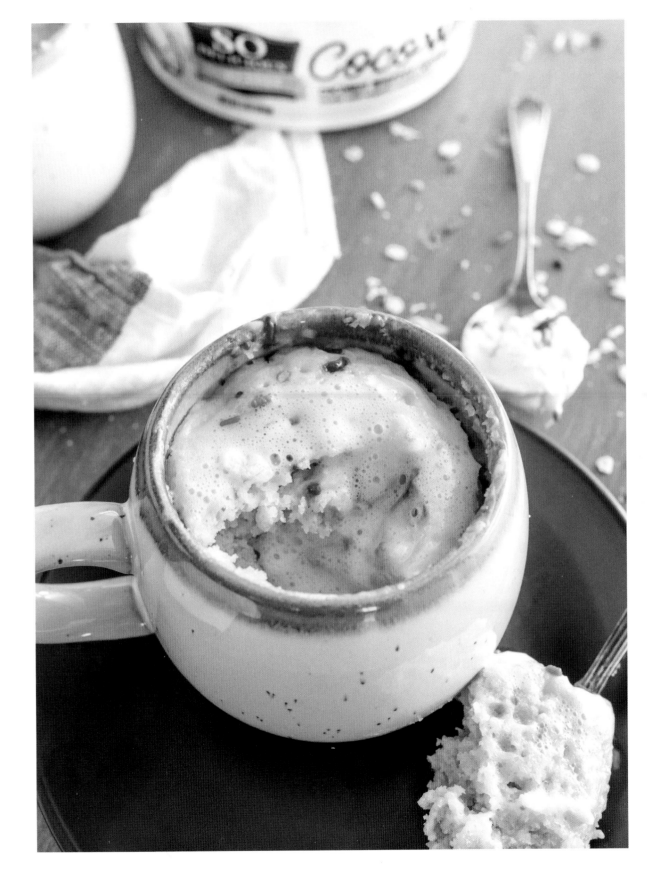

pumpkin zucchini
bread

YIELD: 16 servings
PREP TIME: 10 minutes
COOK TIME: 40 minutes

This bread packs a ton of nutrient- and fiber-rich veggies, yet it tastes like a guilty pleasure. The chocolate chips and walnuts provide both flavor and contrasting texture. Serve the bread with a generous pat of butter with your morning coffee or as a snack or dessert on those cooler fall evenings.

1 cup grated zucchini

3 large eggs, lightly beaten

1½ cups pumpkin puree

1 cup melted coconut oil

1 tablespoon vanilla extract

2½ cups all-purpose flour

1½ cups coconut sugar or granulated sugar

1 teaspoon baking soda

½ teaspoon baking powder

½ teaspoon coarse sea salt

½ teaspoon ground cinnamon

½ teaspoon ground nutmeg

½ teaspoon ground cloves

1 cup chopped raw walnuts

½ cup chocolate chips

1. Preheat the oven to 325°F. Grease a 9-inch square baking pan.

2. Place the grated zucchini in a clean kitchen towel and wring out the excess moisture.

3. In a large bowl, combine the zucchini, eggs, pumpkin puree, coconut oil, and vanilla. In a separate bowl, whisk together the flour, sugar, baking soda, baking powder, salt, and spices until no lumps remain.

4. Incorporate the dry mixture into the wet mixture using a rubber spatula. Fold in the walnuts and chocolate chips. The batter will be thick and sticky; you may need to use your hands to mix the ingredients and melt coconut oil chunks if it solidifies a little.

5. Use the spatula to spread the batter evenly in the prepared pan. Bake until a toothpick inserted into the center comes out clean, 30 to 40 minutes. Let the bread cool completely before cutting into 16 squares.

6. Store in an airtight container on the counter for up to 4 days, or freeze for up to 3 months.

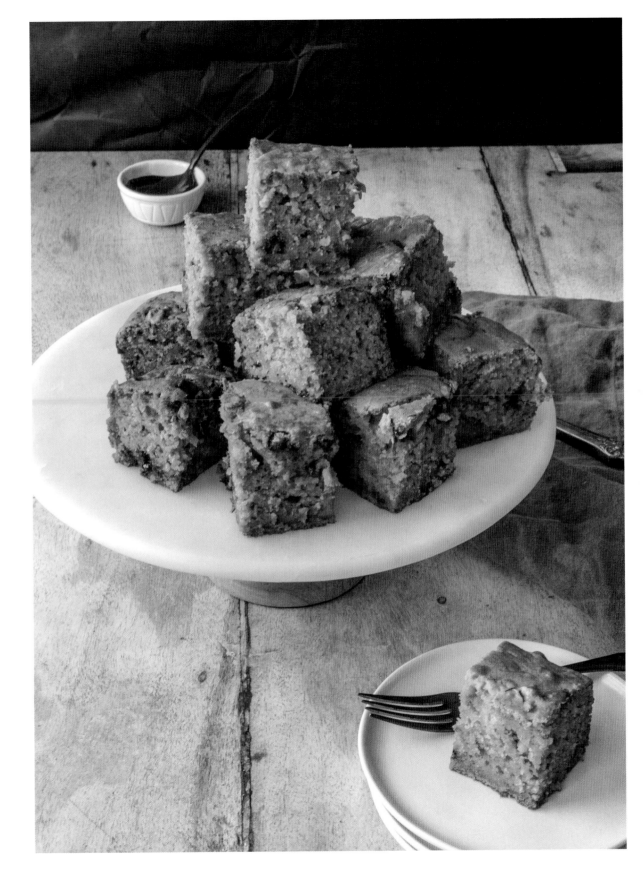

hummus

YIELD: 6 servings
PREP TIME: 10 minutes
COOK TIME: 25 minutes

You will never buy premade hummus again after you try this creamy bean dip, which is great with broccoli or cauliflower florets, carrot sticks, or pita bread. The options are endless! You can also use it to dress sandwiches, eggs, and salads throughout the week.

1 (15-ounce) can chickpeas, drained and rinsed

½ teaspoon baking soda

⅓ cup fresh squeezed lemon juice, or more to taste

2 cloves garlic, roughly chopped

½ teaspoon coarse sea salt

¾ cup tahini, stirred well

2 to 4 tablespoons ice water

½ teaspoon ground cumin

¼ teaspoon paprika, plus more for garnish

2 tablespoons extra-virgin olive oil, plus more for garnish

Chopped fresh parsley or pine nuts, for garnish

1. Place the chickpeas in a medium saucepan and sprinkle with the baking soda. Cover with several inches of water, then bring to a boil over high heat. Lower the heat to medium-high and cook at a low boil for about 20 minutes, until the chickpeas look puffy and most of the skins are falling off. Drain the chickpeas and run cool water over them.

2. Meanwhile, in a food processor or high-powered blender, combine the lemon juice, garlic, and salt. Add the tahini and blend until creamy, stopping to scrape down the sides as necessary.

3. With the food processor or blender running, drizzle in 2 tablespoons of ice water. Scrape down the sides, then continue blending until the mixture is ultra-smooth, pale, and creamy. If it is too thick to blend smoothly, add 1 to 2 tablespoons more ice water.

4. Add the drained chickpeas, cumin, and paprika to the food processor or blender. While blending, drizzle in the oil. Continue blending until the hummus is smooth, about 2 minutes, scraping down the sides as necessary. If the hummus is too thick, add water a tablespoon at a time until the texture is super creamy.

5. Taste and add more salt and/or lemon juice if desired. Transfer to a serving bowl and garnish with a drizzle of oil, a sprinkling of paprika, and parsley or pine nuts.

6. Store in an airtight container in the refrigerator for up to 5 days.

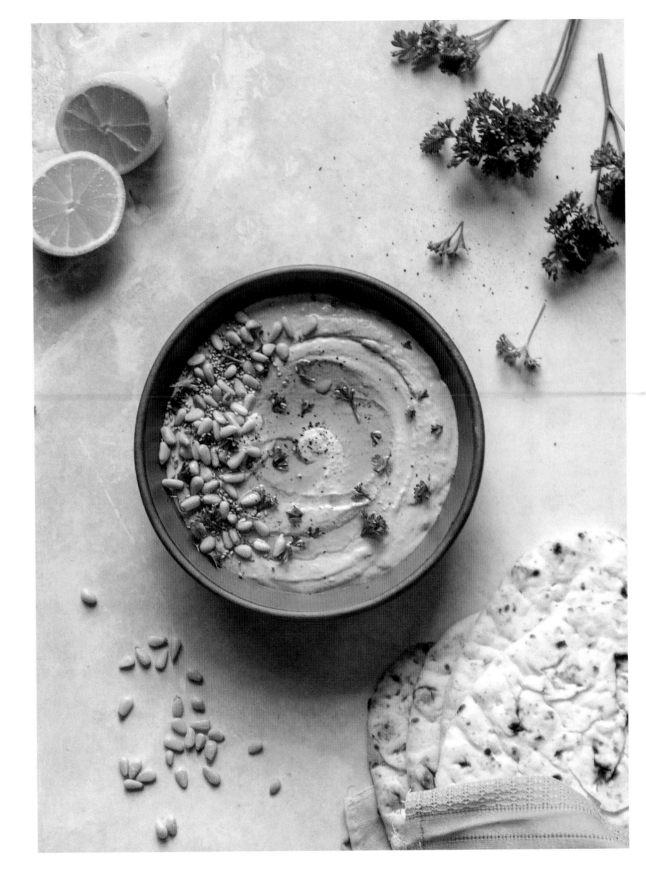

romesco
dip

YIELD: 6 servings
PREP TIME: 15 minutes

This nutty dip is addictive! You can spread it on sandwiches, dip veggies or crackers into it, use it as a dressing or a marinade for meat, or smear it on sourdough for a snack. It is totally plant-based and easy to whip up. If you prefer to roast your own peppers, see page 96.

5 Roma tomatoes, stem end sliced off

3 cloves garlic, minced

2 tablespoons extra-virgin olive oil

1 (12-ounce) jar roasted red peppers, drained

1¼ cups raw almonds

¼ cup chopped fresh parsley

¼ cup stale bread cubes (crusty parts removed)

2 teaspoons coarse sea salt

2 teaspoons ground black pepper

2 tablespoons fresh squeezed lemon juice

1. In a large skillet over medium-high heat, sauté the tomatoes and garlic in the oil until the tomatoes have wrinkled a bit, 8 to 10 minutes. Transfer the tomato mixture to a food processor or high-powered blender and add the remaining ingredients. Blend until you have a coarse puree.

2. Store in an airtight container in the refrigerator for up to 5 days.

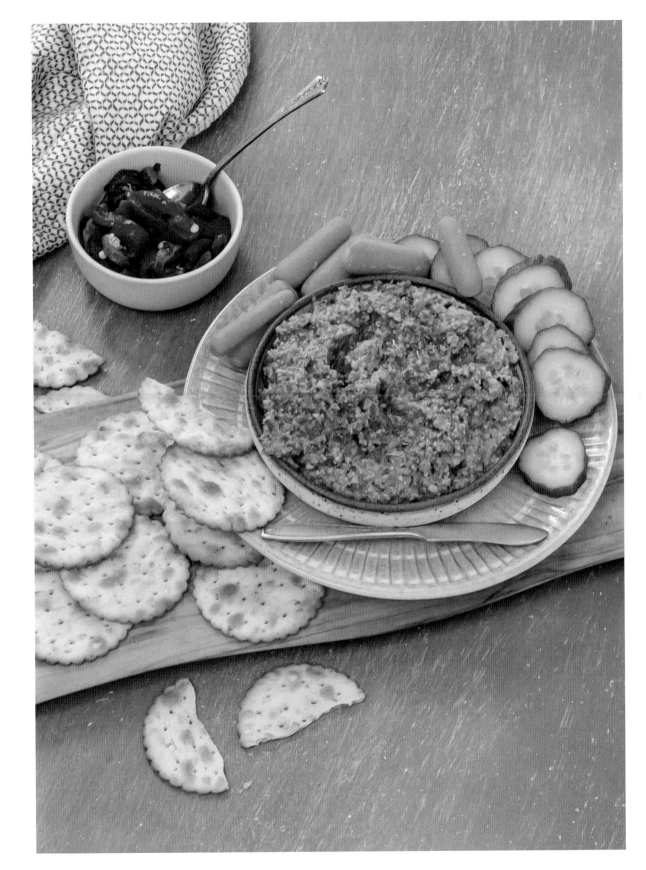

savory
nuts

YIELD: 8 to 10 servings
PREP TIME: 5 minutes
COOK TIME: 15 minutes

These nuts are highly addictive! I recommend portioning them out carefully, or you might find yourself eating the whole batch in one sitting. They have savory notes and are full of herbs, and the cayenne gives them a bit of heat. They take just about twenty minutes to whip up. You can make these in addition to other snacks to help keep you satiated and fueled throughout the week. They also make a great salad topper! I use 1 cup each of raw almonds, cashews, and walnuts, but you can use any nuts in any combinations or ratios you prefer.

1½ tablespoons extra-virgin olive oil

½ teaspoon coconut aminos or soy sauce

½ teaspoon granulated sugar or honey

1 teaspoon garlic powder

1 teaspoon dried rosemary leaves

1 teaspoon dried thyme leaves

½ teaspoon cayenne pepper (optional)

½ teaspoon coarse sea salt

½ teaspoon onion powder

3 cups raw mixed nuts of choice

1. Preheat the oven to 300°F. Line a rimmed baking sheet with parchment paper.

2. In a large bowl, whisk together all the ingredients except the nuts until well combined. Add the nuts and toss until they are evenly coated.

3. Use a rubber spatula to scrape everything in the bowl—the nuts and every bit of the seasoning—onto the prepared baking sheet. Spread the nuts into an even layer. Bake for 8 minutes. Stir and flip the nuts, then continue baking until they are lightly browned, another 7 to 8 minutes. Watch them carefully to make sure they don't burn. Remove from the oven and let the nuts cool and dry on the pan for about 20 minutes.

4. Store in an airtight container for up to a week.

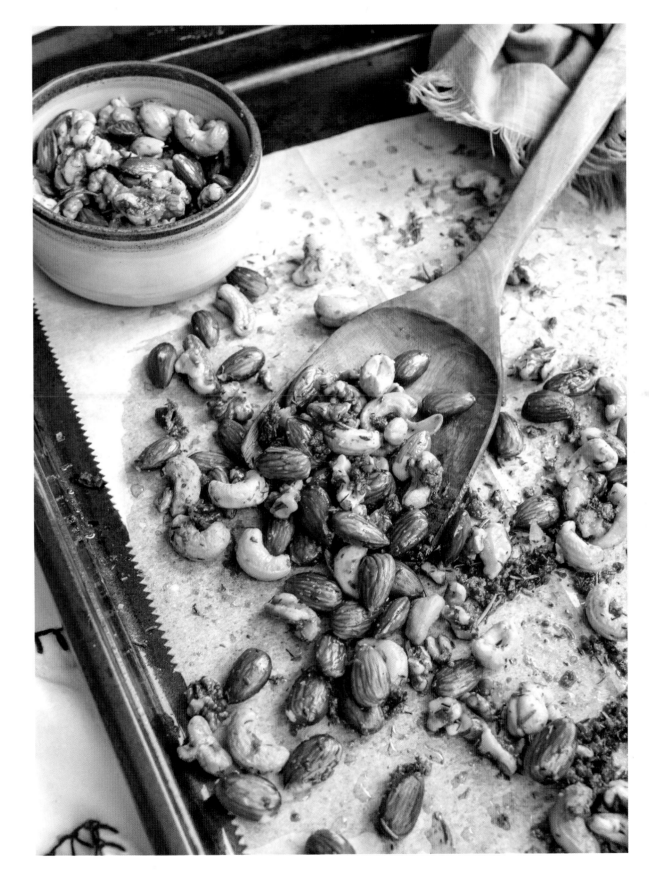

quinoa-stuffed
mushrooms

YIELD: 4 to 6 servings

PREP TIME: 5 minutes (not including time to cook quinoa)

COOK TIME: 25 minutes

You may want to make a double batch of these stuffed mushrooms; they are easy to pop into your mouth and so addictive. They are the healthiest yet tastiest stuffed mushrooms I have ever eaten, and they aren't covered in grease and cheese. I recommend making them ahead of time to have as a ready-to-go snack in the fridge. Heat them up or eat them cold. If you end up with leftovers, they make a great side dish or salad topper.

1 tablespoon extra-virgin olive oil

¼ cup finely chopped onions

2 cloves garlic, minced

1 cup cooked quinoa

1 tablespoon coconut aminos or soy sauce

2 tablespoons vegan sour cream

½ teaspoon paprika

½ teaspoon cayenne pepper (optional)

¼ teaspoon ground black pepper

¼ teaspoon coarse sea salt

1 pound whole baby bella mushrooms

1. Preheat the oven to 350°F. Line a rimmed baking sheet with parchment paper.

2. Heat the oil in a medium skillet over medium-high heat. When hot, add the onions and garlic and sauté until translucent and fragrant, about 2 minutes. Add the quinoa, coconut aminos, sour cream, spices, and salt and stir to combine.

3. Gently pull out the stems of the mushrooms and wipe the insides of the caps with a damp cloth to remove any dirt. Using a spoon, stuff the mushroom caps firmly with the quinoa mixture, being careful not to break them. Place on the prepared baking sheet. Bake for 25 minutes, until the mushrooms are softened, fragrant, and lightly browned.

4. Store in an airtight container in the refrigerator for up to 5 days.

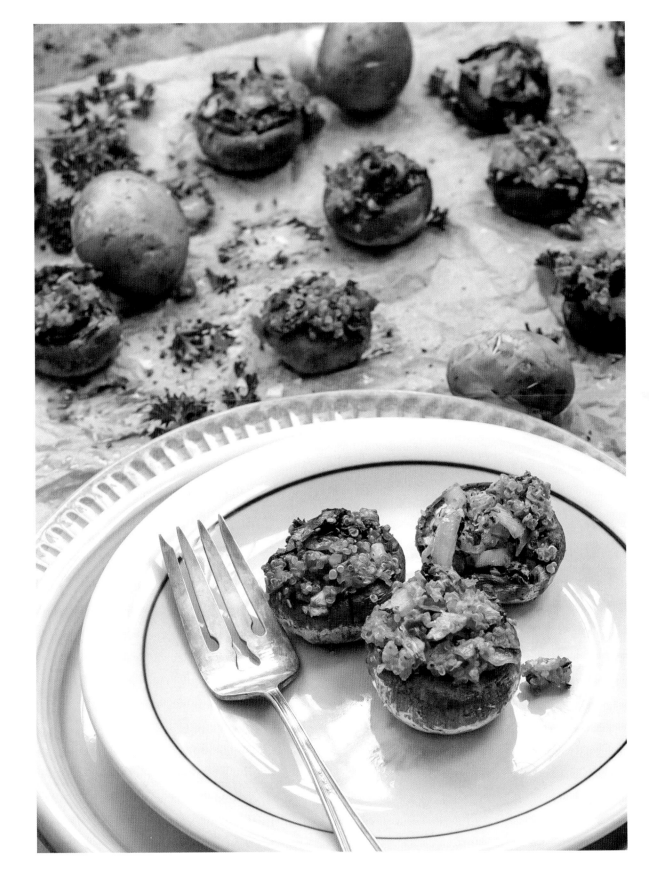

savory herbaceous

popcorn

Many years ago, I went to a vegan pop-up restaurant and had savory popcorn as an appetizer. It had so many delicious flavors in it that I went back for three more servings. Since then, I have refined my taste buds and learned how to create a copycat. Make the popcorn on a Sunday so you can have a savory, herby, cheesy, crunchy plant-based snack to nosh on throughout the week or a great appetizer ready to serve to friends who may drop by.

⅓ cup popcorn kernels, popped, or 8 cups unseasoned prepared popcorn

3 tablespoons nutritional yeast

1 tablespoon garlic powder

1½ teaspoons ground dried thyme

1½ teaspoons dried rosemary leaves

½ teaspoon coarse sea salt

¼ cup coconut oil, melted

Place the popcorn in a gallon-sized zip-top bag. In a small bowl, whisk together the nutritional yeast, garlic powder, thyme, rosemary, and salt. Add the coconut oil to the popcorn in the bag, followed by the seasoning mix. Seal the bag, leaving a little bit of air in it. Gently shake and roll the bag around to evenly coat the popcorn with the seasoning. Store in the bag at room temperature for up to 4 days.

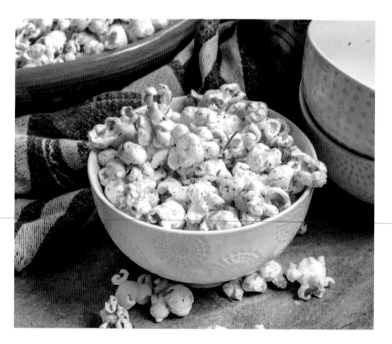

sweet graham cracker

popcorn

YIELD: 8 cups (6 servings)
PREP TIME: 5 minutes

You didn't think I would stop at savory popcorn, did you? I just had to make a sweet popcorn to compete. I know at times we all need some more sweetness in our life. This graham cracker–flavored popcorn isn't overly sweet like most sweetened varieties of popcorn out there, but it's fragrant of cinnamon and so addictive—watch out!

⅓ cup popcorn kernels, popped, or 8 cups unseasoned prepared popcorn

⅓ cup coconut sugar

1½ teaspoons ground cinnamon

¼ teaspoon coarse sea salt

¼ cup coconut oil, melted

Place the popcorn in a gallon-sized zip-top bag. In a small bowl, whisk together the sugar, cinnamon, and salt. Add the coconut oil to the popcorn in the bag, followed by the sugar-cinnamon mixture. Seal the bag, leaving a little bit of air in it. Gently shake and roll the bag around to evenly coat the popcorn with the seasoning. Store in the bag at room temperature for up to 4 days.

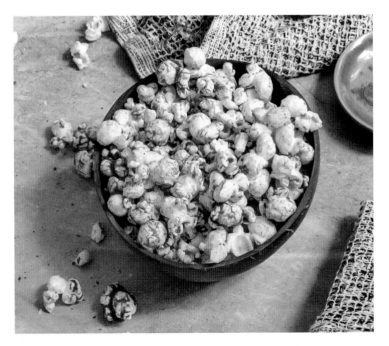

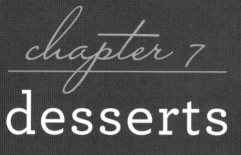

desserts

Vegan Vanilla Cupcakes | 189

Pumpkin Spice Cookies | 192

No-Bake Blondies | 194

Vegan Apple Spice Cake | 196

Peanut Butter Banana Chocolate Chip Bars | 198

Carrot Cake Cookies | 200

Vegan Peanut Butter Cookies | 202

Nutty Payday Bars | 204

Almond Lemon Cookies | 206

Carrot Banana Cupcakes with
Cashew Frosting | 208

vegan vanilla
cupcakes

YIELD: 12 cupcakes
PREP TIME: 10 minutes
COOK TIME: 20 minutes

These cupcakes are perfect for a birthday or special occasion. Your family and friends won't even know they are vegan! The cupcakes go well with my vegan frosting, which is rich and decadent. However, the vanilla cake base is such a versatile canvas, allowing you to pair it with various flavors, so feel free to use any frosting you like.

1 cup SILK unsweetened almond milk

1 teaspoon fresh squeezed lemon juice

1 cup granulated sugar

½ cup extra-light olive oil or canola oil

1 teaspoon vanilla extract

1½ cups all-purpose flour

1½ teaspoons baking powder

½ teaspoon baking soda

¼ teaspoon coarse sea salt

VANILLA FROSTING:

¾ cup vegan butter

¼ cup vegetable shortening

3 to 4 cups powdered sugar

1 teaspoon SILK unsweetened almond milk (if needed)

1. Preheat the oven to 350°F. Line a standard-size 12-cup muffin tin with paper baking cups.

2. In a small bowl, combine the almond milk and lemon juice and let sit for 15 minutes.

3. In a large bowl, beat the sugar, oil, and vanilla with a hand mixer on low to medium speed until well blended into a paste. In a separate bowl, whisk the flour, baking powder, baking soda, and salt to break up any lumps. Add the dry mixture to the wet mixture in small increments, alternating with the milk mixture, until everything is combined. The consistency of the batter should be similar to that of pancake batter.

4. Fill the prepared muffin cups three-quarters full with the batter. Bake for about 20 minutes, until a toothpick inserted into a cupcake comes out clean. Let cool completely in the pan before frosting.

5. While the cupcakes are cooling, make the frosting: Beat the vegan butter and shortening with a hand mixer on medium speed until well combined. Slowly add 3 cups of powdered sugar. Continue to beat on medium-high speed until the frosting is very thick and spreadable. If it is too thin and runny, slowly add up to 1 more cup of powdered sugar; if it is too thick and not spreadable, add the milk.

6. Pipe the frosting onto the cooled cupcakes. Store in an airtight container on the counter for up to 2 days, refrigerate for up to 5 days, or freeze for up to a month.

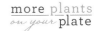

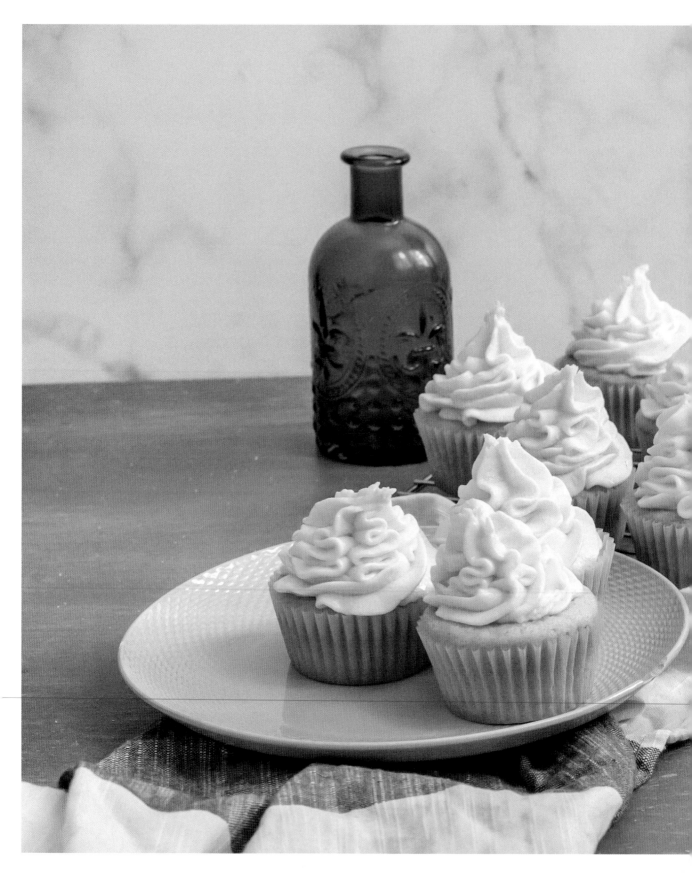

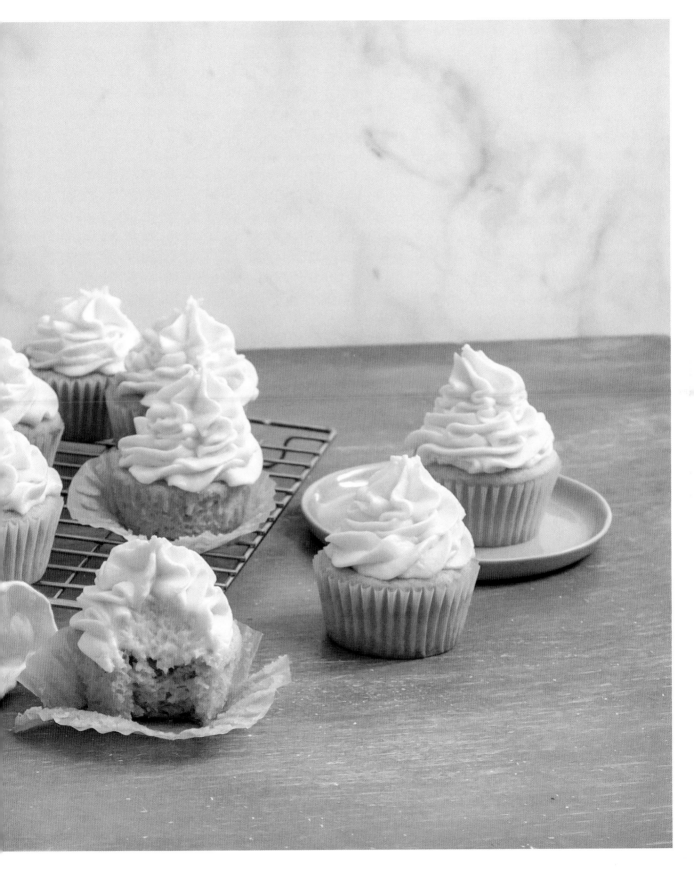

pumkin spice
cookies

YIELD: 14 cookies
PREP TIME: 10 minutes
COOK TIME: 12 minutes

These are the most delicious pumpkin spice cookies I've had—soft, comforting, and full of autumn flavors, with a light icing on top. They are made with real pumpkin and will put you in the mood for fall, although I enjoy them all year long.

1 cup all-purpose flour, or 1½ cups blanched almond flour

1 cup old-fashioned oats

1 tablespoon pumpkin pie spice, plus more for sprinkling

½ teaspoon baking soda

½ teaspoon coarse sea salt

½ teaspoon ground cinnamon

½ cup coconut sugar or granulated sugar

½ cup melted coconut oil

½ cup pumpkin puree

1 teaspoon vanilla extract

1 large egg, room temperature, or 1 flax or chia egg (see page 10)

FROSTING:

½ cup powdered sugar

½ teaspoon SILK unsweetened almond milk, plus more if needed

1. Preheat the oven to 350°F. Line a cookie sheet with parchment paper.

2. In a medium bowl, whisk together the flour, oats, pumpkin pie spice, baking soda, salt, and cinnamon; set aside.

3. In a large bowl, whisk together the sugar and coconut oil until well combined. Whisk in the pumpkin puree, vanilla extract, and egg. Stir in the flour mixture a little at a time to form a soft dough.

4. Form the dough into 1-inch balls and arrange them 2 inches apart on the prepared cookie sheet. Bake until golden, 11 to 12 minutes (or about 16 minutes if using almond flour). Remove from the oven and let cool on the cookie sheet.

5. While the cookies are cooling, make the frosting: In a small bowl, briskly whisk together the powdered sugar and almond milk to form a soft, spreadable frosting. If the mixture is too thick, add more almond milk, ½ teaspoon at a time, to thin it out.

6. Dip the tops of the cookies in the frosting and top with a light sprinkling of pumpkin pie spice.

7. Store in an airtight container on the counter for up to 2 days, refrigerate for up to 5 days, or freeze for up to a month.

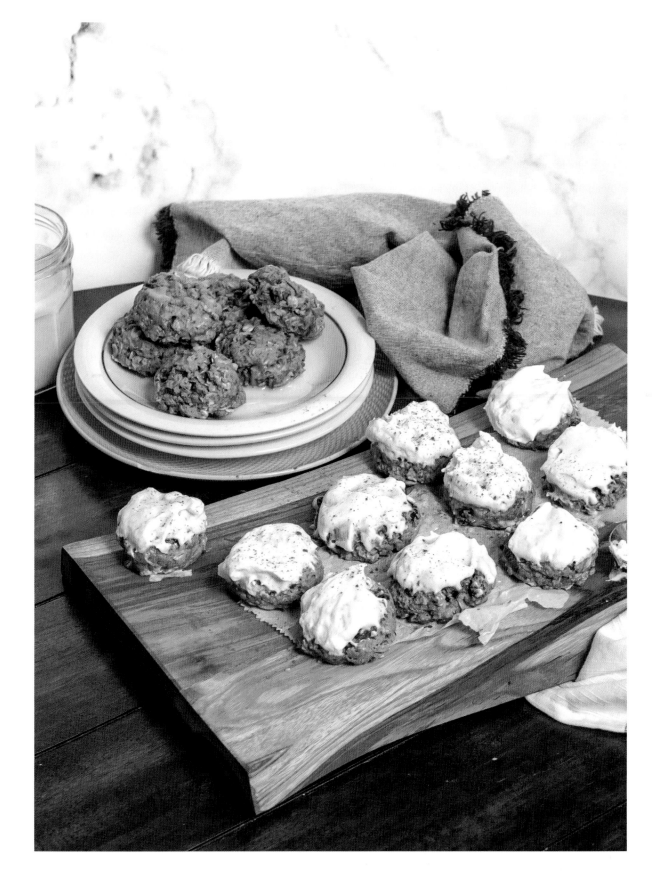

no-bake
blondies

YIELD: 16 squares
PREP TIME: 10 minutes, plus 10 minutes to chill

These no-bake blondies are a favorite in the summer when you don't want to turn on the oven and heat up the kitchen. They are vegan and gluten-free—healthy enough for a midday snack and sweet enough to satisfy that after-dinner sweet tooth.

BASE LAYER:

2 cups blanched almond flour

½ cup almond butter

¼ cup plus 2 tablespoons maple syrup

¼ cup melted coconut oil

2 tablespoons vanilla extract

TOP LAYER:

¾ cup raw walnuts

10 pitted dates

¼ teaspoon coarse sea salt

Maldon sea salt, for sprinkling (optional)

1. Make the base layer: In a large bowl, stir together the almond flour, almond butter, maple syrup, coconut oil, and vanilla. Line a 9 by 5-inch or 8½ by 4½-inch loaf pan with parchment paper and press the mixture evenly into the bottom. Place in the freezer for 10 minutes.

2. Meanwhile, make the top layer: In a food processor, blend the walnuts, dates, and salt until they form a spreadable paste, stopping to scrape the side of the bowl with a rubber spatula as needed.

3. Once the base layer has hardened a bit, gently press the walnut paste on top of the base into an even layer. The paste will be thick and sticky, so you may want to lightly moisten your fingers to make this task a bit easier. Return the pan to the freezer for a few minutes to get the top layer nice and firm.

4. Sprinkle lightly with Maldon salt, if desired. Cut into 16 squares and enjoy. Store in the refrigerator for up to 5 days.

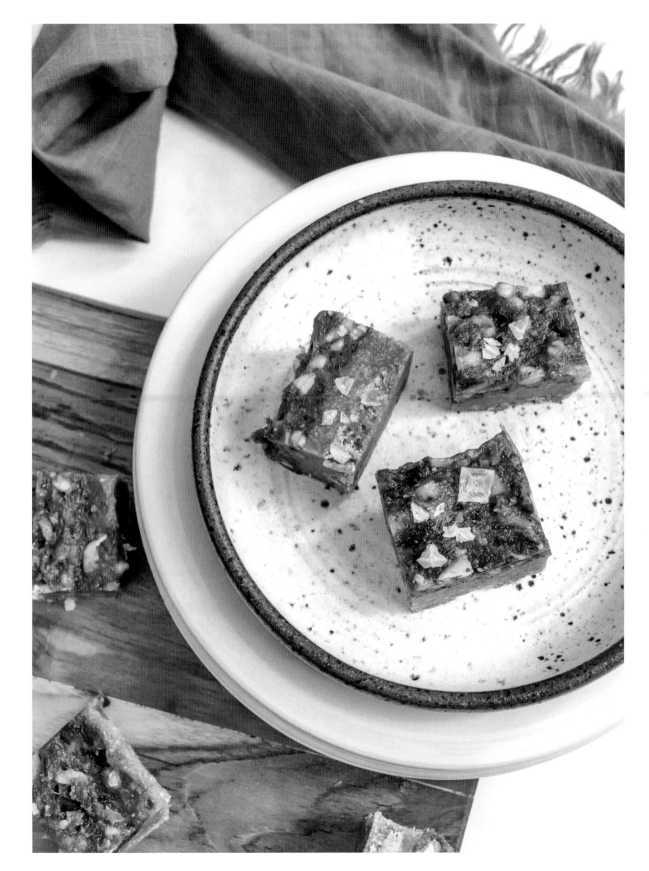

vegan apple spice
cake

YIELD: one single-layer cake
(8 servings)
PREP TIME: 10 minutes
COOK TIME: 30 minutes

This plant-based cake is perfect any time of year, but it is extra special in the fall during peak apple season. You can enjoy it for breakfast without the caramel sauce (note that some brands are not vegan, in case that is important to you), or you can really sweeten it up with a layer of caramel for a special occasion. The choice is yours, and you can't go wrong. You could even double the recipe and make a two-layer cake, as shown.

3 tablespoons grated apple

1½ cups all-purpose flour

1 cup granulated sugar

1¾ teaspoons ground cinnamon

1 teaspoon baking powder

½ teaspoon coarse sea salt

1 cup unsweetened oat milk

¼ cup unsweetened applesauce

1¼ teaspoons apple cider vinegar

2 tablespoons extra-light olive oil or canola oil

1½ teaspoons vanilla extract

¼ cup vegan caramel sauce, store-bought or homemade (page 217) (optional)

¼ cup sliced almonds, for garnish (optional)

1. Preheat the oven to 350°F. Grease a 9-inch springform pan or line it with parchment paper.

2. Place the grated apple in a paper towel or clean kitchen towel and squeeze out the excess liquid.

3. In a medium bowl, whisk together the flour, sugar, cinnamon, baking powder, and salt. In a large bowl, combine the oat milk, applesauce, vinegar, oil, vanilla, and grated apple.

4. Add the dry ingredients to the wet ingredients and mix well. Pour the batter into the prepared pan and smooth the top. Bake until a toothpick inserted into the center comes out clean, 25 to 30 minutes. Let the cake cool completely in the pan.

5. Run a butter knife between the cake and the edge of the pan. Gently release the springform ring and transfer the cake to a platter. If desired, spread the caramel sauce on top and garnish with the sliced almonds.

6. Store in an airtight container on the counter for up to 2 days, refrigerate for up to 5 days, or freeze for up to a month.

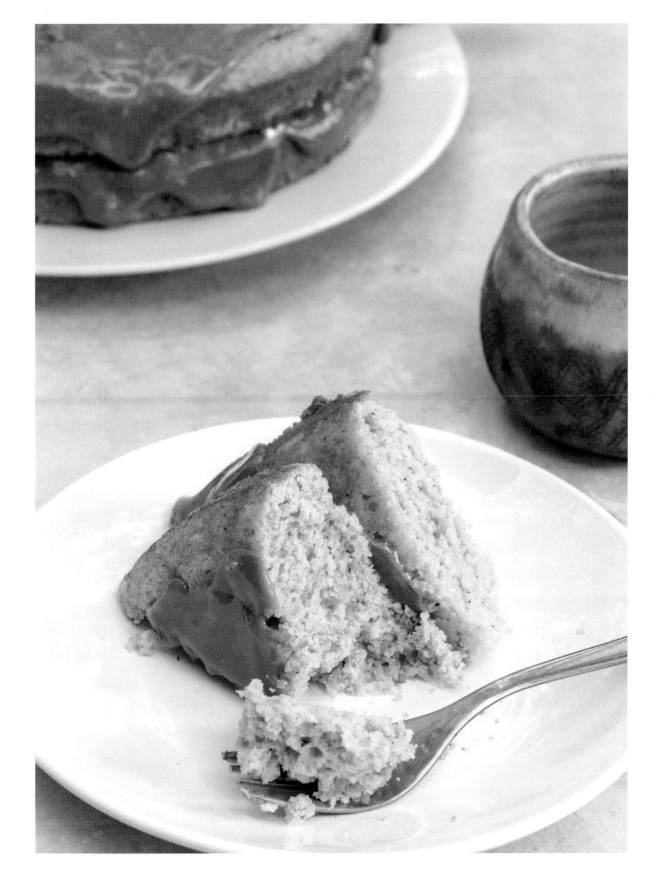

peanut butter banana
chocolate chip bars

YIELD: 12 bars
PREP TIME: 10 minutes
COOK TIME: 20 minutes

Can you think of a better combo than banana, chocolate, and peanut butter? These bars are perfect for breakfast or as a healthy dessert. They are fluffy like cake and have a slight crust on the top like a brownie. They are very popular in my house.

2 to 3 overripe bananas

⅓ cup granulated sugar

¼ cup natural creamy peanut butter

3 tablespoons melted coconut oil

2 tablespoons SILK unsweetened almond milk

1 large egg, room temperature

1 teaspoon vanilla or almond extract

¾ cup all-purpose flour

½ teaspoon ground cinnamon

½ teaspoon baking soda

⅛ teaspoon coarse sea salt

⅓ cup chocolate chips

½ cup crushed walnuts (optional)

1. Preheat the oven to 350°F. Grease an 8-inch square baking pan or line it with parchment paper.

2. In a large bowl, mash the bananas with a fork, then measure out exactly 1 cup; reserve any extra for another use or discard. Add the sugar, peanut butter, coconut oil, almond milk, egg, and extract and whisk until smooth.

3. In another bowl, whisk together the flour, cinnamon, baking soda, and salt. Slowly add the dry ingredients to the wet ingredients and mix with a rubber spatula or wooden spoon. Do not overmix! Fold in the chocolate chips and the nuts, if using.

4. Spread the batter in the prepared pan. Bake until a toothpick inserted into the center comes out clean, 16 to 20 minutes. Remove from the oven and let cool completely before cutting into 12 bars.

5. Store in an airtight container on the counter for up to 4 days, or freeze for up to 3 months.

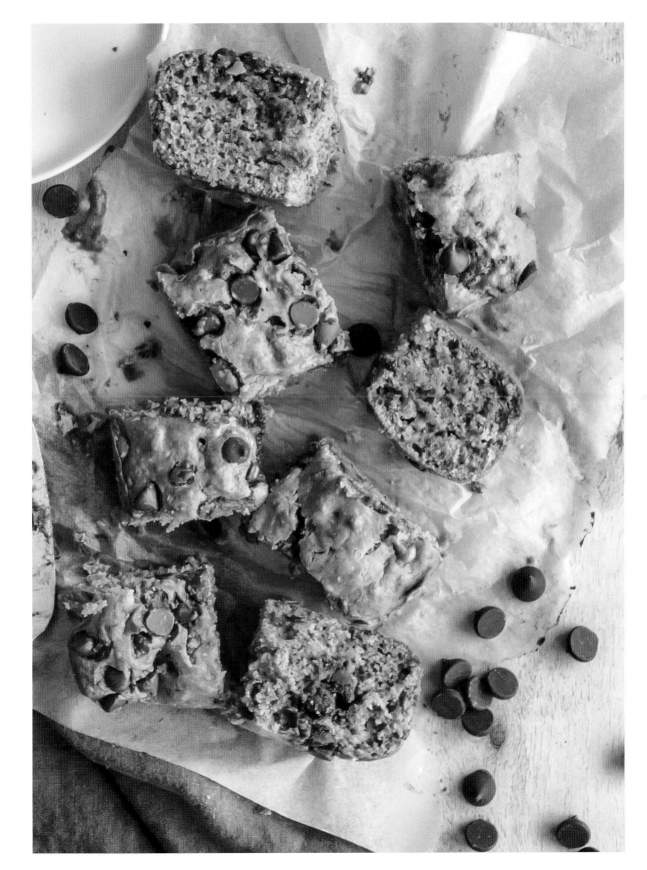

carrot cake
cookies

These soft, chewy cookies are sweet and decadent and will wow your friends and family. Using a food processor to grate the carrots makes the process go much faster, but you can also grate them by hand using a cheese grater. If you don't want to take the time to make the glaze, you can dip your cookies in So Delicious CocoWhip for an extra-special flavorful treat.

1 cup all-purpose flour

1 cup muesli or old-fashioned oats

1 teaspoon baking soda

1½ teaspoons ground cinnamon

⅛ teaspoon ground nutmeg

¼ cup melted coconut oil

⅓ cup coconut sugar or granulated sugar

¼ cup granulated sugar

1 large egg, room temperature

2 teaspoons vanilla extract

1 cup grated carrots

¼ cup chopped raw walnuts

¼ cup raisins (optional)

GLAZE (OPTIONAL):

¼ cup powdered sugar

1 to 2 tablespoons SILK unsweetened almond milk or water

1. Preheat the oven to 350°F. Line two cookie sheets with parchment paper.

2. In a medium bowl, whisk together the flour, muesli, baking soda, cinnamon, and nutmeg. In a large bowl, whisk together the oil, sugars, egg, and vanilla until smooth. Stir in the carrots, walnuts, and raisins, if using. Add the dry mixture to the wet in small increments, mixing well after each addition.

3. Using a 1-tablespoon measuring spoon, drop the dough onto one of the prepared baking sheets, spacing the cookies about 2 inches apart. Bake until slightly browned, about 11 minutes. Transfer the cookies to a cooling rack to cool completely. Repeat with the remaining dough and the second cookie sheet.

4. Meanwhile, make the glaze: In a small bowl, whisk together the powdered sugar and 1 tablespoon of the almond milk until smooth. If it's too thick to drizzle, whisk in the remaining 1 tablespoon of milk, a teaspoon at a time.

5. Drizzle the glaze over the cooled cookies using a spoon or the tines of a fork. (Alternatively, you can put the glaze in a small plastic bag, snip off a tiny corner of the bag, and pipe the glaze over the cookies.)

6. Store in an airtight container on the counter for up to 2 days, refrigerate for up to 5 days, or freeze for up to a month.

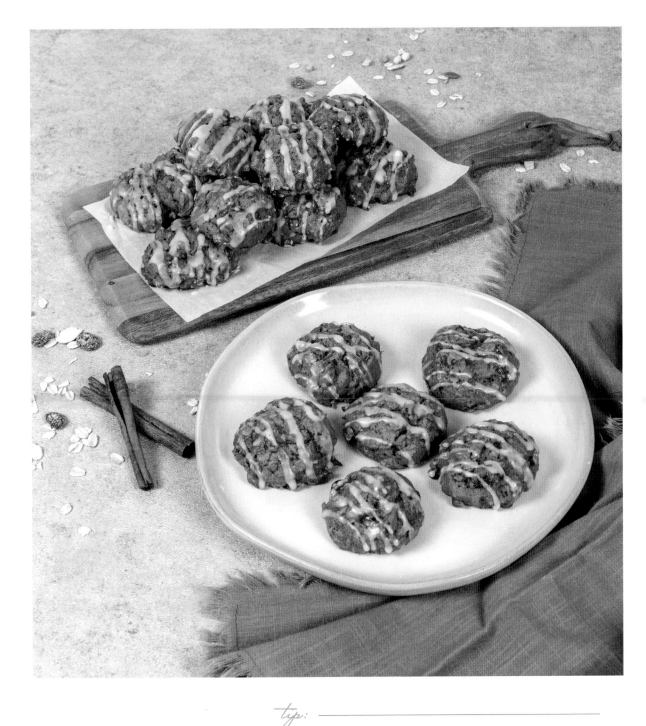

tip: —————————————————————————————————

To make the cookies gluten-free, simply swap out the
all-purpose flour for gluten-free 1:1 flour. To make them
fully plant-based, use a chia or flax egg (see page 10) in
place of the egg.

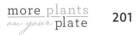

vegan peanut butter
cookies

YIELD: 14 to 16 cookies
PREP TIME: 5 minutes
COOK TIME: 9 to 12 minutes

These cookies are for the ultimate peanut butter lover. The almond flour not only makes the cookies grain- and gluten-free but also gives them a wonderful chewy texture. If you prefer softer cookies, bake them for slightly less time; for crispier cookies, bake them a few minutes longer.

1 cup natural peanut butter

⅓ cup SILK unsweetened almond milk

2 teaspoons vanilla extract

¾ cup coconut sugar or granulated sugar

1¼ cups blanched almond flour

¼ teaspoon coarse sea salt

Maldon sea salt, for sprinkling (optional)

1. Preheat the oven to 350°F. Line a cookie sheet with parchment paper.

2. In a large bowl, use a wooden spoon to stir together the peanut butter, almond milk, and vanilla until smooth. Add the sugar and stir until no lumps remain. In a separate bowl, whisk together the almond flour and coarse salt. Incorporate the almond flour mixture into the peanut butter mixture. The dough will be very thick, so you may need to use your hands to mix everything until well blended and free of lumps.

3. Form the dough into 1-inch balls and arrange them 2 inches apart on the prepared cookie sheet. Bake for 9 to 10 minutes for chewier cookies or 11 to 12 minutes for crispier cookies.

4. Sprinkle Maldon salt over the cookies while they're still hot, if desired, then let them cool and set completely on the cookie sheet before serving. Store in an airtight container on the counter for up to 4 days, or freeze for up to 3 months.

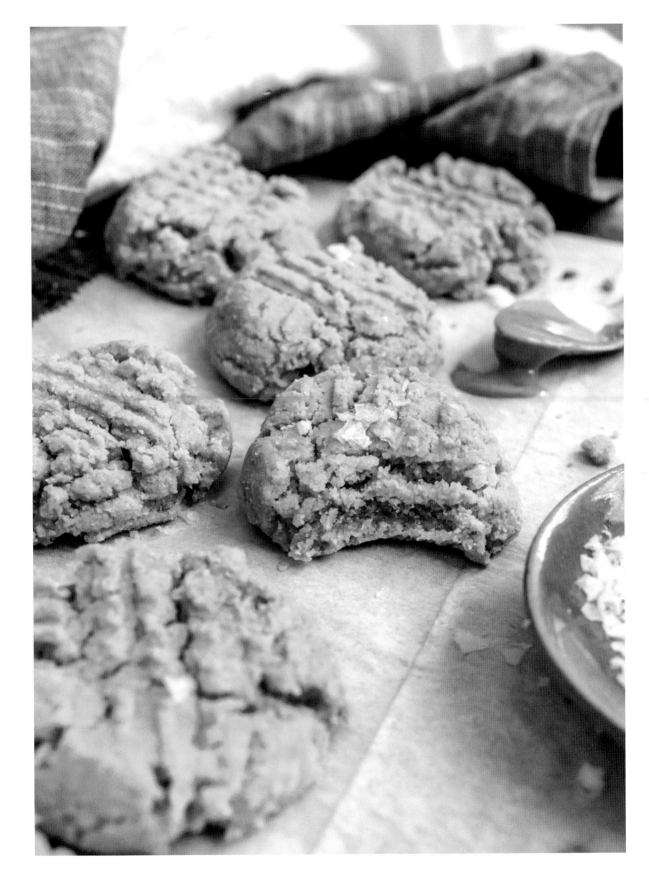

nutty
payday bars

YIELD: 12 small bars
PREP TIME: 15 minutes, plus 45 minutes to chill
COOK TIME: 20 minutes

These melt-in-your-mouth vegan morsels are a freezer treat, so you can easily prepare them for desserts or snacks throughout the week. You can make them with almond butter or another type of nut butter if you have a peanut allergy; substitute stevia or monkfruit sweetener for the sugar if you are watching your sugar intake.

CAKE LAYER:

½ cup vegan butter

2 cups blanched almond flour

¼ cup arrowroot starch or cornstarch

½ cup granulated sugar

MAPLE PEANUT BUTTER FUDGE LAYER:

1 cup natural peanut butter or nut butter of choice

¼ cup melted coconut oil

2½ tablespoons maple syrup

¼ teaspoon coarse sea salt

1 cup chopped raw peanuts (optional)

For the cake layer:

1. Preheat the oven to 350°F. Line an 8½ by 4½-inch loaf pan or similar-sized pan with parchment paper, leaving some paper overhanging the sides.

2. In a stand mixer, or in a large bowl with a hand mixer, cream the butter, flour, arrowroot, and sugar. Press the mixture into the prepared pan, making the top as even as possible.

3. Bake the cake layer for about 20 minutes, until lightly browned and firm. Let cool completely on the counter.

For the maple peanut butter fudge layer:

4. In a large bowl, stir together the peanut butter, coconut oil, maple syrup, and salt.

5. Pour the peanut butter mixture over the cooled cake layer and smooth the top. Sprinkle with the peanuts, if using. Freeze for at least 45 minutes. Once set, take the pan out of the freezer and carefully lift the two layers out of the pan using the overhanging parchment paper. Cut into 12 small bars.

6. Store in a resealable plastic bag or other freezer-safe container in the freezer for up to 3 months. Eat directly from the freezer or allow to thaw for about 2 minutes for a softer bar.

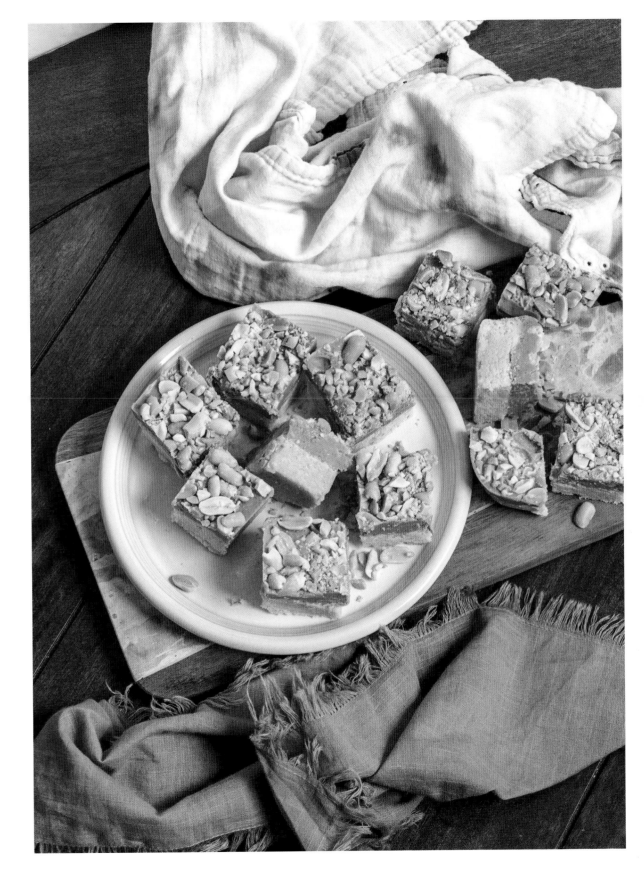

almond lemon
cookies

YIELD: <u>10 cookies</u>

PREP TIME: <u>10 minutes, plus 1 hour to chill dough</u>

COOK TIME: <u>13 minutes</u>

These zesty, soft and chewy cookies are perfect for a midday snack or an after-dinner treat and pair nicely with a cup of tea. The almond extract makes them taste much sweeter than they are.

½ cup coconut sugar or granulated sugar

¼ cup melted coconut oil

Grated zest and juice of 1 lemon

1 large egg, room temperature

1 large egg yolk, room temperature

½ teaspoon almond extract (optional)

1½ cups all-purpose flour

1 teaspoon baking powder

⅛ teaspoon coarse sea salt

¼ cup sliced almonds

¼ cup powdered sugar, for topping (optional)

1. In a large bowl, mix together the sugar, oil, lemon zest and juice, egg, egg yolk, and almond extract, if using, with a wooden spoon. In a separate bowl, whisk together the flour, baking powder, salt, and almonds. Stir the dry mixture into the wet ingredients, making sure the flour is fully incorporated. Use your hands to form the dough into a ball.

2. Wrap the dough ball in plastic wrap and place in the refrigerator to chill for at least 1 hour.

3. When ready to bake the cookies, preheat the oven to 350°F and line a cookie sheet with parchment paper.

4. Scoop tablespoon-sized balls of the chilled dough (I use an ice cream scoop). If using the powdered sugar, put it on a plate and roll the balls in the sugar to coat. (You also have the option to sprinkle the cookies with the sugar after baking for a different look.)

5. Place the balls on the prepared cookie sheet, spaced about 1 inch apart; they will spread only a little. Bake for 11 to 13 minutes, until lightly browned on top.

6. Store in an airtight container on the counter for up to 4 days, or freeze for up to 3 months.

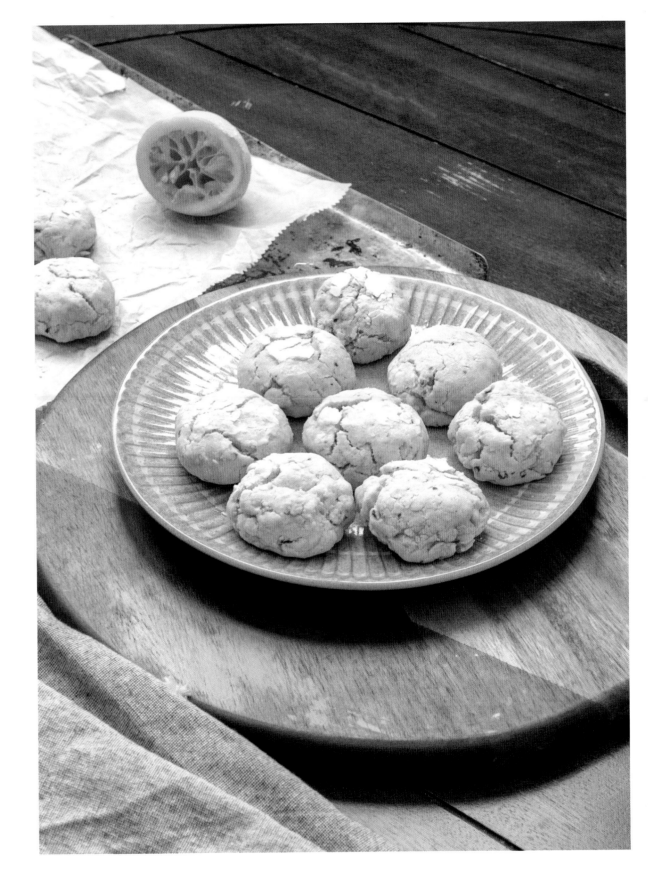

carrot banana cupcakes
with cashew frosting

YIELD: 12 cupcakes
PREP TIME: 10 minutes
COOK TIME: 20 minutes

These cupcakes are like a mash-up of the classic carrot cake and banana bread. The creamy vanilla-scented cashew frosting makes them even more delicious and decadent. You can also skip the frosting and serve them as breakfast muffins.

CUPCAKES:

1 cup all-purpose flour

¾ cup granulated sugar

1 teaspoon ground cinnamon

½ teaspoon ground nutmeg

1 teaspoon baking soda

Pinch of coarse sea salt

2 overripe bananas, mashed

1½ cups grated carrots

⅔ cup melted coconut oil

2 large eggs, lightly beaten

CASHEW FROSTING:

1 cup raw cashews, soaked in very hot water for at least 1 hour (up to overnight) and drained

3 tablespoons SILK unsweetened almond milk

2 tablespoons maple syrup

½ teaspoon vanilla extract

2 tablespoons powdered sugar

¼ teaspoon arrowroot starch or cornstarch

1. Preheat the oven to 350° F. Line a standard-size 12-cup muffin tin with paper baking cups.

2. Combine the flour, sugar, cinnamon, nutmeg, baking soda, and salt in a medium bowl.

3. In a large bowl, combine the mashed bananas, grated carrots, and oil; reserve about a tablespoon of the carrots for garnish, if desired. Fold the dry mixture into the wet mixture; do not overmix. Add the beaten eggs and stir a few times more with a rubber spatula. It's important to not overmix the batter.

4. Scoop the batter into the prepared muffin tin, filling each cup halfway or a little less. Bake for 15 to 20 minutes, until a toothpick inserted into the center of a cupcake comes out clean. Let cool completely in the pan before frosting.

5. While the cupcakes are cooling, make the frosting: Put the cashews in a high-powered blender or food processor and blend well. Add the almond milk, maple syrup, vanilla, powdered sugar, and arrowroot; blend until creamy and smooth.

6. Pipe the frosting onto the cooled cupcakes. Garnish with the reserved grated carrots, if desired. Store in the refrigerator for up to 5 days.

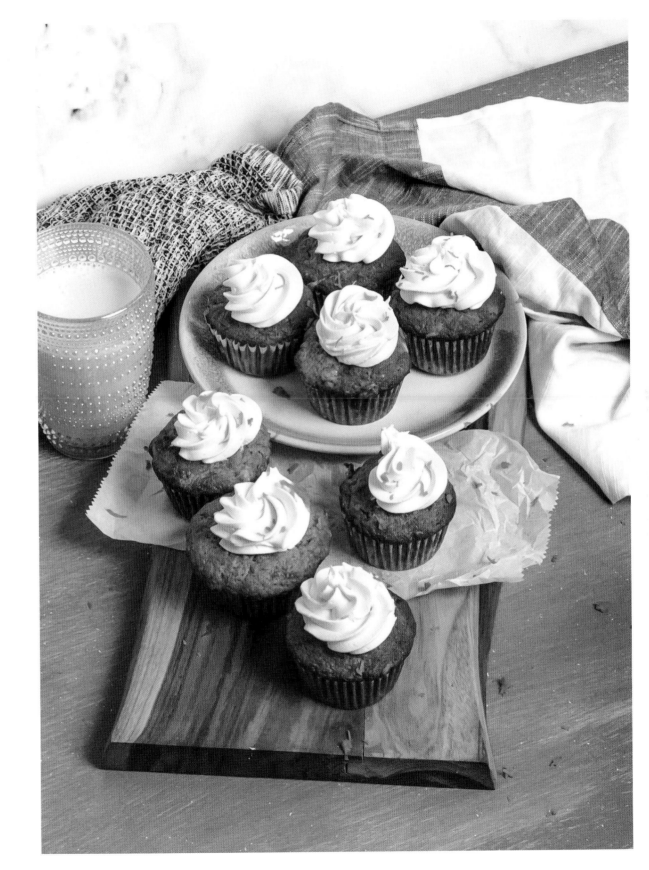

chapter 8

sauces & more

Teriyaki Sauce | 211

Plant-Based Parmesan | 212

Cilantro Chimichurri | 213

Cashew Queso | 214

Magic Garlic Sauce or Dressing | 216

Plant-Based Caramel Sauce | 217

teriyaki

sauce

YIELD: 2 cups
PREP TIME: 8 minutes
COOK TIME: about 15 minutes

1¼ cups water, divided

¼ cup packed brown sugar

¼ cup soy sauce

1½ tablespoons honey

2 cloves garlic, minced

½ teaspoon ginger powder

2 tablespoons arrowroot starch or cornstarch

2 to 3 tablespoons white sesame seeds (optional)

1½ teaspoons red pepper flakes (optional)

Teriyaki sauce is so versatile. In this book, it's used in my Teriyaki Salmon Sheet Pan Dinner recipe (page 148), but it's also great on chicken or pork.

1. In a medium saucepan, combine 1 cup of the water, the brown sugar, soy sauce, honey, garlic, and ginger powder. Bring to a gentle boil over medium heat.

2. In a small bowl, whisk the arrowroot with the remaining ¼ cup of water to make a slurry. Whisk the slurry into the contents of the saucepan. Lower the head and simmer, stirring occasionally, until the sauce reaches your desired thickness. If it becomes too thick, add more water to thin it out.

3. Remove from the heat and stir in the sesame seeds and/ or red pepper flakes, if using. Whisk well before serving. Store in an airtight container in the fridge for up to 4 days.

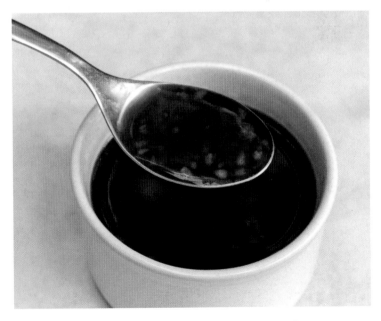

plant-based

parmesan

YIELD: about 1¾ cups
PREP TIME: 5 minutes

I first made this recipe when I was in my early twenties. I have since perfected it—the secret is to add more garlic powder and oregano! I always have a jar of plant-based parm in my fridge. I promise you, it is the perfect vegan swap for Parmesan cheese. You are more than welcome to use the real stuff; however, if you want to have a few fully plant-based meals throughout the week, this is a terrific mix to add to salads, pastas, pizzas—basically anything savory. I even eat it by the spoonful for a snack!

1 cup raw cashew pieces

¼ cup plus 1 tablespoon nutritional yeast

1 teaspoon garlic powder

½ teaspoon ground dried oregano

½ teaspoon coarse sea salt

¼ teaspoon onion powder

Put all the ingredients in a food processor or high-powered blender. Pulse until the cashews are crushed into tiny bits and the mixture resembles grated Parmesan cheese. Store in an airtight container in the fridge for up to 2 weeks.

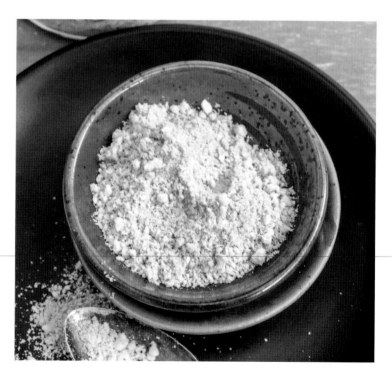

cilantro
chimichurri

YIELD: 1 cup
PREP TIME: 8 minutes

Chimichurri sounds complicated and fancy, but it's the easiest way to use up extra herbs in the fridge and offers a powerhouse of flavors. You can use it to top salmon or veggies or dip fries into it.

1 cup roughly chopped fresh cilantro

1 cup roughly chopped fresh parsley

⅓ cup roughly chopped red onions

3 cloves garlic, roughly chopped

1½ teaspoons roughly chopped jalapeño pepper

1 teaspoon Italian seasoning

1 teaspoon coarse sea salt

1 teaspoon ground black pepper

½ teaspoon red pepper flakes, or more to taste

¾ cup extra-virgin olive oil

¼ cup fresh lime juice, or more to taste

Put all the ingredients in a high-powered blender and pulse until smooth with just a little bit of texture. Taste and add more red pepper flakes or lime juice, if desired. Pour the sauce into a tightly sealed jar or container. It will keep in the refrigerator for up to 4 days. Be sure to shake the jar before using, as the oil will separate.

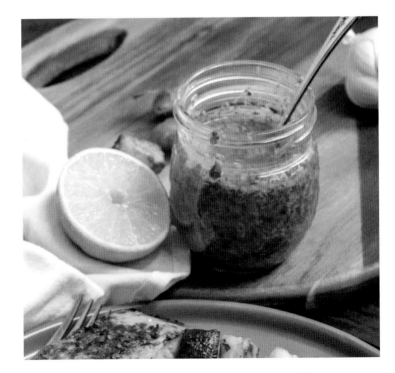

cashew

queso

YIELD: 1½ cups
PREP TIME: 10 minutes
COOK TIME: 2 minutes

1 cup raw cashew pieces

¾ cup water

½ cup nutritional yeast

¼ cup drained diced tomatoes and green chiles (such as Ro-Tel)

2 cloves garlic, peeled

1 teaspoon chili powder

¼ teaspoon coarse sea salt

FOR TOPPING (OPTIONAL):

Diced avocado

Diced fresh tomatoes

Finely chopped fresh parsley or cilantro

You probably won't miss heavy dairy-based queso once you nail this recipe! Every queso lover who has tried it has been impressed. Cashews usually need to be soaked for hours to get them soft enough to achieve a creamy consistency, but I have mastered a way to soften them quickly. This sauce can be made in just minutes!

1. Combine the cashews and water in a small microwave-safe bowl. Microwave on high for 1 minute. Let cool completely, then microwave on high for 1 more minute.

2. Transfer the cashews and warm water to a high-powered blender. Add the nutritional yeast, tomatoes and chiles, garlic cloves, chili powder, and salt and blend until smooth. Add some hot water if needed to achieve the consistency of whipping cream. Pour into a bowl and top with avocado, fresh tomatoes and/or parsley, if using. Dip away!

3. This queso is best enjoyed fresh but will keep in the refrigerator for up to 4 days. It will thicken in the fridge; if needed, add a little water to thin it out again. To reheat, microwave for about 1 minute. It scorches easily, so keep an eye on it.

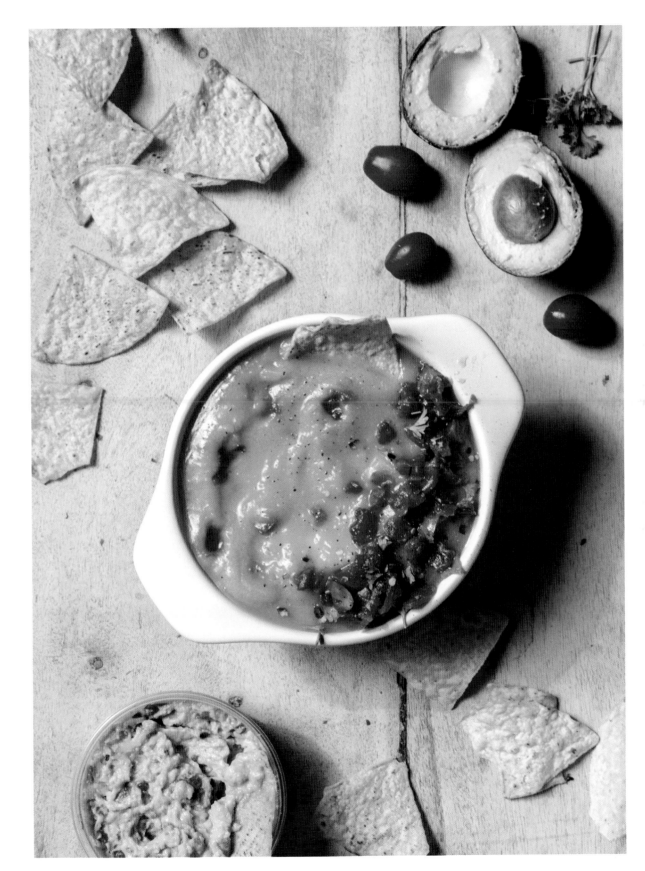

magic garlic sauce
or dressing

YIELD: 1½ cups
PREP TIME: 5 minutes

Be forewarned: this sauce is addictive. Similar to hummus (see page 178 for my recipe), it works great over salads, with fries, on pizzas, in pasta dishes—you name it! I prefer the mellow undertones of roasted garlic in this magic sauce, but you can easily use raw garlic; just be aware that your sauce will have a spicier garlic bite to it.

½ cup canned chickpeas, drained and rinsed

¼ cup plus 1 tablespoon water

3 to 4 cloves roasted or raw garlic (see Tip)

2 tablespoons fresh squeezed lemon juice

1 tablespoon extra-virgin olive oil

¼ teaspoon honey

¼ teaspoon coarse sea salt

Put all the ingredients in a food processor or high-powered blender and pulse until well blended. Taste and add more salt if needed. Add more water a tablespoon at a time if you desire a thinner, dressing-like consistency. Store in an airtight container in the refrigerator for up to 4 days.

tip:

To roast garlic, peel the desired number of cloves (or use a whole bulb, unpeeled), then drizzle lightly with olive oil, wrap in foil, and place in a 350°F oven for about 10 minutes, until fragrant and slightly browned.

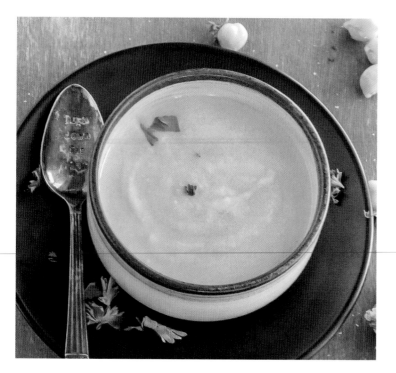

plant-based
caramel sauce

YIELD: ½ cup
PREP TIME: 2 minutes
COOK TIME: 3 minutes

¼ cup coconut oil

¼ cup maple syrup

1½ tablespoons smooth
almond butter

1 teaspoon vanilla extract

This thick, amber-colored caramel sauce is hands down the best treat I have made to date—plus it's almost too easy to be true. It is hard to find store-bought caramel that is free of dairy and other animal products, so you will want to save this recipe.

In a small saucepan, bring the coconut oil and maple syrup to a gentle simmer over medium-low heat. Cook, whisking well, for about 2 minutes, until the mixture starts to darken. Turn off the heat and whisk in the almond butter and vanilla. Continue whisking until all the ingredients are fully melted; the sauce will thicken as it cools. Store in an airtight container in the refrigerator for up to 4 days. To reheat, microwave on low power for about 30 seconds.

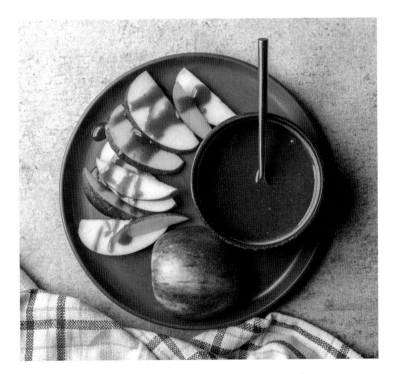

index

A

acorn squash
    Chipotle Acorn Squash & Kale Stew, 76–77
    Harvest Salad with Maple Vinaigrette, 154–155
all-purpose flour, swap for, 32
almond butter
    Blueberry Breakfast Cookies, 37
    Maple Almond Baked Oatmeal, 60–61
    No-Bake Blondies, 194–195
    No-Bake Trail Mix Bars, 172–173
    Plant-Based Caramel Sauce, 217
    Strawberry Bliss Balls, 169
Almond Cashew Coconut Chicken Tenders with Honey Mustard, 122–123
Almond Lemon Cookies, 206–207
almond milk
    Broccoli Cheese Twice-Baked Potatoes, 74–75
    Carrot Banana Cupcakes with Cashew Frosting, 208–209
    Carrot Breakfast Cake, 62–63
    Carrot Cake Cookies, 200–201
    Creamy Fettuccine with Avocado, 90–91
    Mushroom Stroganoff, 80–81
    Pan-Fried Chicken & Veggies with Rosemary Gravy, 136–137
    Peanut Butter Banana Chocolate Chip Bars, 198–199
    Plant-Based Tuscan Alfredo with Artichokes & Mushrooms, 146–147
    Pumpkin Spice Cake, 62–63
    Pumpkin Spice Cookies, 192–193
    Vegan Peanut Butter Cookies, 202–203
    Vegan Vanilla Cupcakes, 189–191
almonds
    Almond Cashew Coconut Chicken Tenders with Honey Mustard, 122–123
    Almond Lemon Cookies, 206–207
    Cranberry Almond Granola, 56–57
    Maple Almond Baked Oatmeal, 60–61
    No-Bake Trail Mix Bars, 172–173
    Romesco Dip, 180–181
    Vegan Apple Spice Cake, 196–197
aluminum foil, 16
Apple Blueberry Baked Oatmeal, 52–53
apples
    about, 25
    Apple Blueberry Baked Oatmeal, 52–53
    Harvest Salad with Maple Vinaigrette, 154–155
    Vegan Apple Spice Cake, 196–197
artichoke hearts
    Artichoke Zucchini Pasta with Roasted Red Pepper Sauce, 96–97
    Plant-Based Tuscan Alfredo with Artichokes & Mushrooms, 146–147
    Zoodles with Artichoke Pesto & Mushrooms, 72–73
Artichoke Zucchini Pasta with Roasted Red Pepper Sauce, 96–97
arugula
    Sweet Potato Tacos, 144–145
avocado oil, 28
avocados
    about, 25
    Breakfast Burritos, 54–55
    Broccoli Potato Hash, 64–65
    Cashew Queso, 214–215
    Cauliflower Hash, 46–47
    Chicken Sausage Fajitas, 124–125
    Chicken Tacos, 108–109
    Creamy Fettuccine with Avocado, 90–91
    Fiesta Salad with Plant-Based Ranch, 156–157
    HBE Breakfast Salad, 44–45
    Loaded Black Bean Quesadillas, 82–83
    Mushroom & Spinach Enchiladas with Cashew Queso, 94–95
    Plant-Based Creamy Broccoli Casserole, 86–87
    Roasted Veggie Salad, 158–159
    Shrimp Cobb Salad, 160–161
    Superfood Salad with Lemon Honey Dressing, 152–153
    Veggie Egg Cups, 38–39

B

Bacon & Egg Casserole, 58–59
Baked Falafel-Style Balls, 98–99
baked goods, adding vegetables to, 10
Baked Spiced Cauliflower, 151
Baked Ziti, 106–107
bananas
    about, 25
    Blueberry Banana Bread, 170–171
    Blueberry Breakfast Cookies, 37
    Carrot Banana Cupcakes with Cashew Frosting, 208–209
    Carrot Breakfast Cake, 62–63
    Gluten-Free Protein Pancakes, 40–41
    Maple Almond Baked Oatmeal, 60–61
    Maple Vanilla Overnight Oats, 42–43
    Peanut Butter Banana Chocolate Chip Bars, 198–199
    Pumpkin Spice Cake, 62–63
basil
    Artichoke Zucchini Pasta with Roasted Red Pepper Sauce, 96–97
    marinara sauce, 70–71
    Mushroom & Brussels Sprouts Pizza, 140–141
    Pepperoni Rigatoni, 126–127
    Zoodles with Artichoke Pesto & Mushrooms, 72–73
beans, 28. *See also specific types*
beef
    Baked Ziti, 106–107
    Beef Spaghetti Squash with Tzatziki, 128–129
    Sunday Burgers, 142–143
Beef Spaghetti Squash with Tzatziki, 128–129
bell peppers
    Artichoke Zucchini Pasta with Roasted Red Pepper Sauce, 96–97
    Bacon & Egg Casserole, 58–59
    Beef Spaghetti Squash with Tzatziki, 128–129
    Breakfast Burritos, 54–55
    Cauliflower Curry, 78–79

Cauliflower Hash, 46–47
Chicken Sausage Fajitas, 124–125
Chicken Tacos, 108–109
Hard-Boiled Egg Plate with
    Roasted Veggies, 50–51
Shredded BBQ Chicken &
    Peppers, 120–121
Stuffed Peppers, 112–113
Turkey Veggie Meatballs, 104–105
Veggie Egg Cups, 38–39
black beans
    Fiesta Salad with Plant-Based
        Ranch, 156–157
    Loaded Black Bean Quesadillas,
        82–83
    Sweet Potato Burgers, 84–85
    Three-Bean Turkey Chili, 114–115
    Veggie Taco Bowls, 67–69
blueberries
    about, 25
    Apple Blueberry Baked Oatmeal,
        52–53
    Blueberry Banana Bread, 170–171
    Blueberry Breakfast Cookies, 37
    Maple Vanilla Overnight Oats,
        42–43
Blueberry Banana Bread, 170–171
Blueberry Breakfast Cookies, 37
bread/breadcrumbs
    Baked Falafel-Style Balls, 98–99
    Plant-Based Creamy Broccoli
        Casserole, 86–87
    Portobello Mushroom Burgers
        with Broccoli Slaw, 88–89
    Romesco Dip, 180–181
    Sneaky Turkey Meatloaf, 110–111
    Sunday Burgers, 142–143
    Sweet Potato Burgers, 84–85
    Zucchini Parm Boats, 70–71
Breakfast Burritos, 54–55
broccoli
    about, 25
    Breakfast Burritos, 54–55
    Broccoli Cheese Twice-Baked
        Potatoes, 74–75
    Broccoli Potato Hash, 64–65
    Chicken & Veggie Sheet Pan
        Meal, 118–119
    Garlic Dijon Chicken, 101–103
    HBE Breakfast Salad, 44–45
    Maple Bourbon Salmon with
        Veggie Rice & Broccoli,
        133–135
    Plant-Based Creamy Broccoli
        Casserole, 86–87
    Portobello Mushroom Burgers
        with Broccoli Slaw, 88–89
    Roasted Veggie Salad, 158–159

Broccoli Cheese Twice-Baked
    Potatoes, 74–75
Broccoli Potato Hash, 64–65
brown rice. See rice
brown sugar
    Teriyaki Sauce, 211
Brussels sprouts
    Harvest Salad with Maple
        Vinaigrette, 154–155
    Mushroom & Brussels Sprouts
        Pizza, 140–141
    Peanut Butter Brussels Sprouts,
        166–167
    Teriyaki Salmon Sheet Pan
        Dinner, 148–149
butter, swap for, 32

C

cabbage
    Plant-Based Creamy Broccoli
        Casserole, 86–87
cakes. See also cupcakes
    Carrot Breakfast Cake, 62–63
    Oatmeal Funfetti Mug Cake,
        174–175
    Pumpkin Spice Cake, 62–63
    Vegan Apple Spice Cake, 196–197
Carrot Banana Cupcakes with
    Cashew Frosting, 208–209
Carrot Breakfast Cake, 62–63
Carrot Cake Cookies, 200–201
carrots
    Carrot Banana Cupcakes with
        Cashew Frosting, 208–209
    Carrot Breakfast Cake, 62–63
    Carrot Cake Cookies, 200–201
    Stuffed Peppers, 112–113
    Sweet Potato Burgers, 84–85
Cashew Queso, 214–215
    HBE Breakfast Salad, 44–45
    Mushroom & Spinach Enchiladas
        with Cashew Queso, 94–95
    Turkey Veggie Tacos, 130–131
cashews
    Almond Cashew Coconut
        Chicken Tenders with Honey
        Mustard, 122–123
    Carrot Banana Cupcakes with
        Cashew Frosting, 208–209
    Cashew Queso, 214–215
    Plant-Based Parmesan, 212
cauliflower
    Baked Spiced Cauliflower, 151
    Cauliflower Curry, 78–79
    Cauliflower Hash, 46–47
    Hard-Boiled Egg Plate with
        Roasted Veggies, 50–51
    Roasted Veggie Salad, 158–159

Cauliflower Curry, 78–79
Cauliflower Hash, 46–47
cheddar cheese
    Broccoli Cheese Twice-Baked
        Potatoes, 74–75
cheese. See also specific types
    Breakfast Burritos, 54–55
    substitution for, 32
    Sunday Burgers, 142–143
chia seeds
    about, 28
    Carrot Breakfast Cake, 62–63
    Maple Almond Baked Oatmeal,
        60–61
    Maple Vanilla Overnight Oats,
        42–43
    Pumpkin Spice Cake, 62–63
chicken
    Almond Cashew Coconut
        Chicken Tenders with Honey
        Mustard, 122–123
    Chicken Tacos, 108–109
    Chicken & Veggie Sheet Pan
        Meal, 118–119
    Garlic Dijon Chicken, 101–103
    Pan-Fried Chicken & Veggies
        with Rosemary Gravy, 136–137
    roasting with vegetables, 10
    Shredded BBQ Chicken &
        Peppers, 120–121
    swap for, 32
    Turkey Veggie Meatballs, 104–105
Chicken Sausage Fajitas, 124–125
Chicken Tacos, 108–109
Chicken & Veggie Sheet Pan Meal,
    118–119
chickpeas
    Hummus, 178–179
    Magic Garlic Sauce, 216
Chipotle Acorn Squash & Kale
    Stew, 76–77
chocolate
    No-Bake Trail Mix Bars, 172–173
    Peanut Butter Banana Chocolate
        Chip Bars, 198–199
    Pumpkin Zucchini Bread, 176–177
cilantro
    Cilantro Chimichurri, 213
    Turkey Feta Meatballs with Red
        Pepper Sauce, 116–117
Cilantro Chimichurri recipe, 213
coconut
    Almond Cashew Coconut
        Chicken Tenders with Honey
        Mustard, 122–123
    Strawberry Bliss Balls, 169
coconut aminos
    about, 28

coconut aminos (continued)
  Almond Cashew Coconut
    Chicken Tenders with Honey
    Mustard, 122–123
  Portobello Mushroom Burgers
    with Broccoli Slaw, 88–89
  Quinoa-Stuffed Mushrooms,
    184–185
  Savory Nuts, 182–183
  Sweet Potato Tacos, 144–145
coconut milk
  Apple Blueberry Baked Oatmeal,
    52–53
  Cauliflower Curry, 78–79
  Maple Almond Baked Oatmeal,
    60–61
  Maple Vanilla Overnight Oats,
    42–43
  Oatmeal Funfetti Mug Cake,
    174–175
  Plant-Based Protein Waffles,
    48–49
coconut milk creamer
  about, 27
  Artichoke Zucchini Pasta with
    Roasted Red Pepper Sauce,
    96–97
  Pan-Fried Chicken & Veggies
    with Rosemary Gravy, 136–137
  Plant-Based Creamy Broccoli
    Casserole, 86–87
  Plant-Based Tuscan Alfredo with
    Artichokes & Mushrooms,
    146–147
coconut yogurt. See also yogurt
  Apple Blueberry Baked Oatmeal,
    52–53
  Broccoli Cheese Twice-Baked
    Potatoes, 74–75
coleslaw mix
  Portobello Mushroom Burgers
    with Broccoli Slaw, 88–89
cookies and bars
  Almond Lemon Cookies, 206–207
  Blueberry Breakfast Cookies, 37
  Carrot Cake Cookies, 200–201
  No-Bake Blondies, 194–195
  No-Bake Trail Mix Bars, 172–173
  Nutty Payday Bars, 204–205
  Peanut Butter Banana Chocolate
    Chip Bars, 198–199
  Pumpkin Spice Cookies, 192–193
  Vegan Peanut Butter Cookies,
    202–203
corn
  Chicken Tacos, 108–109
  Fiesta Salad with Plant-Based
    Ranch, 156–157

Loaded Black Bean Quesadillas,
    82–83
  Veggie Taco Bowls, 67–69
corn tortillas. See tortillas
cranberries
  Cranberry Almond Granola,
    56–57
  No-Bake Trail Mix Bars, 172–173
  Peanut Butter Brussels Sprouts,
    166–167
Cranberry Almond Granola, 56–57
Creamy Fettuccine with Avocado,
    90–91
cucumbers
  Beef Spaghetti Squash with
    Tzatziki, 128–129
  Superfood Salad with Lemon
    Honey Dressing, 152–153
cupcakes. See also cakes
  Carrot Banana Cupcakes with
    Cashew Frosting, 208–209
  Vegan Vanilla Cupcakes, 189–191

D
dates
  No-Bake Blondies, 194–195
  Strawberry Bliss Balls, 169
dietary restrictions, 32
dill
  Beef Spaghetti Squash with
    Tzatziki, 128–129
  Fiesta Salad with Plant-Based
    Ranch, 156–157
dips
  Hummus, 178–179
  Romesco Dip, 180–181

E
eggs
  about, 27
  Bacon & Egg Casserole, 58–59
  Breakfast Burritos, 54–55
  Hard-Boiled Egg Plate with
    Roasted Veggies, 50–51
  HBE Breakfast Salad, 44–45
  mixing vegetables with, 10
  Shrimp Cobb Salad, 160–161
  substitution for, 32
  Veggie Egg Cups, 38–39
equipment, for meal prep, 15–17

F
feta cheese
  Broccoli Cheese Twice-Baked
    Potatoes, 74–75
  Turkey Feta Meatballs with Red
    Pepper Sauce, 116–117

fettuccine. See pasta
Fiesta Salad with Plant-Based
    Ranch, 156–157
fish. See salmon; shrimp
flax seeds
  about, 28
  Carrot Breakfast Cake, 62–63
  Maple Almond Baked Oatmeal,
    60–61
flour tortillas. See tortillas
food allergies, 32
fruits, 25–26. See also specific types

G
garlic
  about, 26
  Garlic Dijon Chicken, 101–103
  Magic Garlic Sauce, 216
  roasting, 216
Garlic Dijon Chicken, 101–103
ginger
  Cauliflower Curry, 78–79
  Teriyaki Salmon Sheet Pan
    Dinner, 148–149
Gluten-Free Protein Pancakes,
    40–41
goat cheese
  Baked Ziti, 106–107
  Broccoli Cheese Twice-Baked
    Potatoes, 74–75
  Sunday Burgers, 142–143
  Veggie Egg Cups, 38–39
granola
  Blueberry Banana Bread, 170–171
  Cranberry Almond Granola,
    56–57
  as a snack, 30
Greek yogurt. See yogurt
green chilies
  Cashew Queso, 214–215
  Chicken Tacos, 108–109
  Loaded Black Bean Quesadillas,
    82–83
  Three-Bean Turkey Chili, 114–115
green onions
  Broccoli Cheese Twice-Baked
    Potatoes, 74–75
  Cauliflower Hash, 46–47
  Teriyaki Salmon Sheet Pan
    Dinner, 148–149
grocery shopping, 23–31

H
Hard-Boiled Egg Plate with Roasted
    Veggies, 50–51
Harvest Salad with Maple
    Vinaigrette, 154–155

HBE Breakfast Salad, 44–45
hemp hearts
    Maple Vanilla Overnight Oats,
        42–43
herbs, 24–25. *See also specific types*
honey
    Almond Cashew Coconut
        Chicken Tenders with Honey
        Mustard, 122–123
    Apple Blueberry Baked Oatmeal,
        52–53
    Cranberry Almond Granola,
        56–57
    Fiesta Salad with Plant-Based
        Ranch, 156–157
    Magic Garlic Sauce, 216
    Savory Nuts, 182–183
    Superfood Salad with Lemon
        Honey Dressing, 152–153
    Teriyaki Sauce, 211
    Turkey Feta Meatballs with Red
        Pepper Sauce, 116–117
hot sauce
    Shredded BBQ Chicken &
        Peppers, 120–121
hummus
    as a snack, 30
    recipe, 178–179

I–J
ingredients
    pantry staples, 23–31
    tips for choosing, 11
jalapeño peppers
    Cilantro Chimichurri, 213
    Loaded Black Bean Quesadillas,
        82–83
    Pepperoni Rigatoni, 126–127
    Three-Bean Turkey Chili, 114–115

K
kale
    Chipotle Acorn Squash & Kale
        Stew, 76–77
    Harvest Salad with Maple
        Vinaigrette, 154–155
    HBE Breakfast Salad, 44–45
    Superfood Salad with Lemon
        Honey Dressing, 152–153
kidney beans
    Chipotle Acorn Squash & Kale
        Stew, 76–77
    Three-Bean Turkey Chili, 114–115

L
leafy greens, 9. *See also* lettuce
leftovers, storing, 21

lemons
    Almond Lemon Cookies, 206–207
    Beef Spaghetti Squash with
        Tzatziki, 128–129
    Creamy Fettucine with Avocado,
        90–91
    Fiesta Salad with Plant-Based
        Ranch, 156–157
    Hummus, 178–179
    Magic Garlic Sauce, 216
    Mediterranean Red Pepper
        Risotto with Shrimp, 138–139
    Pan-Fried Chicken & Veggies
        with Rosemary Gravy, 136–137
    Shrimp Cobb Salad, 160–161
    Superfood Salad with Lemon
        Honey Dressing, 152–153
    Turkey Feta Meatballs with Red
        Pepper Sauce, 116–117
    Vegan Vanilla Cupcakes, 189–191
    Zoodles with Artichoke Pesto &
        Mushrooms, 72–73
    Zucchini Lasagna with Plant-
        Based Ricotta, 92–93
Lesser Evil Clean Snacks, 31
lettuce. *See also* mixed greens
    Chicken Sausage Fajitas, 124–125
    Portobello Mushroom Burgers
        with Broccoli Slaw, 88–89
    Shredded BBQ Chicken &
        Peppers, 120–121
    Shrimp Cobb Salad, 160–161
    Sunday Burgers, 142–143
    Sweet Potato Burgers, 84–85
    Turkey Veggie Tacos, 130–131
    Veggie Taco Bowls, 67–69
limes
    Cauliflower Curry, 78–79
    Chicken & Veggie Sheet Pan
        Meal, 118–119
    Cilantro Chimichurri, 213
    Fiesta Salad with Plant-Based
        Ranch, 156–157
    Veggie Taco Bowls, 67–69
Loaded Black Bean Quesadillas,
    82–83

M
Magic Garlic Sauce, 216
Maple Almond Baked Oatmeal,
    60–61
Maple Bourbon Salmon with
    Veggie Rice & Broccoli, 133–135
maple syrup
    Apple Blueberry Baked Oatmeal,
        52–53
    Carrot Banana Cupcakes with
        Cashew Frosting, 208–209

Cranberry Almond Granola,
    56–57
Harvest Salad with Maple
    Vinaigrette, 154–155
Maple Almond Baked Oatmeal,
    60–61
Maple Bourbon Salmon with
    Veggie Rice & Broccoli, 133–135
Maple Vanilla Overnight Oats,
    42–43
No-Bake Blondies, 194–195
No-Bake Trail Mix Bars, 172–173
Nutty Payday Bars, 204–205
Oatmeal Funfetti Mug Cake,
    174–175
Plant-Based Caramel Sauce, 217
Portobello Mushroom Burgers
    with Broccoli Slaw, 88–89
Strawberry Bliss Balls, 169
Maple Vanilla Overnight Oats,
    42–43
marinara sauce
    Baked Ziti, 106–107
    Pepperoni Rigatoni, 126–127
    Zucchini Lasagna with Plant-
        Based Ricotta, 92–93
    Zucchini Parm Boats, 70–71
mayonnaise
    Portobello Mushroom Burgers
        with Broccoli Slaw, 88–89
meal prepping, tips for, 12–22
meat, storing, 18, 19. *See also
    specific types*
meatballs/meatloaf, mixing
    vegetables into, 10
Mediterranean Red Pepper Risotto
    with Shrimp, 138–139
milk/milk alternatives, 27
miso paste
    about, 29
    Fiesta Salad with Plant-Based
        Ranch, 156–157
mixed greens
    Fiesta Salad with Plant-Based
        Ranch, 156–157
    HBE Breakfast Salad, 44–45
    Roasted Veggie Salad, 158–159
mozzarella cheese
    Mushroom & Brussels Sprouts
        Pizza, 140–141
    Stuffed Peppers, 112–113
    Zucchini Lasagna with Plant-
        Based Ricotta, 92–93
    Zucchini Parm Boats, 70–71
Mushroom & Brussels Sprouts
    Pizza, 140–141
Mushroom & Spinach Enchiladas
    with Cashew Queso, 94–95

Mushroom Stroganoff, 80–81
mushrooms
 about, 25
 Baked Falafel-Style Balls, 98–99
 Baked Ziti, 106–107
 Beef Spaghetti Squash with
  Tzatziki, 128–129
 Maple Bourbon Salmon with
  Veggie Rice & Broccoli,
  133–135
 Mushroom & Brussels Sprouts
  Pizza, 140–141
 Mushroom & Spinach Enchiladas
  with Cashew Queso, 94–95
 Mushroom Stroganoff, 80–81
 Plant-Based Tuscan Alfredo with
  Artichokes & Mushrooms,
  146–147
 Portobello Mushroom Burgers
  with Broccoli Slaw, 88–89
 Quinoa-Stuffed Mushrooms,
  184–185
 Stuffed Peppers, 112–113
 Three-Bean Turkey Chili, 114–115
 Turkey Veggie Meatballs, 104–105
 Turkey Veggie Tacos, 130–131
 Zoodles with Artichoke Pesto &
  Mushrooms, 72–73
 Zucchini Lasagna with Plant-
  Based Ricotta, 92–93
mustard
 Almond Cashew Coconut
  Chicken Tenders with Honey
  Mustard, 122–123
 Fiesta Salad with Plant-Based
  Ranch, 156–157
 Garlic Dijon Chicken, 101–103
 Maple Bourbon Salmon with
  Veggie Rice & Broccoli,
  133–135
 Shrimp Cobb Salad, 160–161
 Sneaky Turkey Meatloaf, 110–111

N
No-Bake Blondies, 194–195
No-Bake Trail Mix Bars, 172–173
noodles. See also pasta
 Mushroom Stroganoff, 80–81
nut butter. See also specific types
 Nutty Payday Bars, 204–205
 as a snack, 31
nutritional yeast
 Cashew Queso, 214–215
 Plant-Based Parmesan, 212
 Plant-Based Tuscan Alfredo with
  Artichokes & Mushrooms,
  146–147
 Savory Herbaceous Popcorn, 186

Zucchini Lasagna with Plant-
 Based Ricotta, 92–93
nuts. See also specific types
 about, 29
 Savory Nuts, 182–183
Nutty Payday Bars, 204–205

O
oat milk
 Creamy Fettuccine with Avocado,
  90–91
 Vegan Apple Spice Cake, 196–197
Oatmeal Funfetti Mug Cake,
 174–175
oats
 about, 29
 Apple Blueberry Baked Oatmeal,
  52–53
 Baked Falafel-Style Balls, 98–99
 Blueberry Breakfast Cookies, 37
 Carrot Breakfast Cake, 62–63
 Carrot Cake Cookies, 200–201
 Cranberry Almond Granola,
  56–57
 Maple Almond Baked Oatmeal,
  60–61
 Maple Vanilla Overnight Oats,
  42–43
 No-Bake Trail Mix Bars, 172–173
 Oatmeal Funfetti Mug Cake,
  174–175
 Pumpkin Spice Cake, 62–63
 Pumpkin Spice Cookies, 192–193
 Sneaky Turkey Meatloaf, 110–111
 Strawberry Bliss Balls, 169
 Turkey Feta Meatballs with Red
  Pepper Sauce, 116–117
olive oil, 28
olives
 Mediterranean Red Pepper
  Risotto with Shrimp, 138–139
onions, 26

P
Pan-Fried Chicken & Veggies with
 Rosemary Gravy, 136–137
Parmesan cheese
 Artichoke Zucchini Pasta with
  Roasted Red Pepper Sauce,
  96–97
 Chipotle Acorn Squash & Kale
  Stew, 76–77
 Creamy Fettuccine with Avocado,
  90–91
 Parsnip Fries, 164–165
 Sweet Potato Fries with
  Parmesan, 162–163

Zoodles with Artichoke Pesto &
 Mushrooms, 72–73
Zucchini Parm Boats, 70–71
Parsnip Fries, 164–165
pasta. See also noodles
 Artichoke Zucchini Pasta with
  Roasted Red Pepper Sauce,
  96–97
 Baked Ziti, 106–107
 Creamy Fettuccine with Avocado,
  90–91
 Pepperoni Rigatoni, 126–127
 Plant-Based Tuscan Alfredo with
  Artichokes & Mushrooms,
  146–147
peanut butter
 Nutty Payday Bars, 204–205
 Peanut Butter Banana Chocolate
  Chip Bars, 198–199
 Peanut Butter Brussels Sprouts,
  166–167
 as a snack, 31
 swap for, 32
 Vegan Peanut Butter Cookies,
  202–203
Peanut Butter Banana Chocolate
 Chip Bars, 198–199
Peanut Butter Brussels Sprouts,
 166–167
pecans
 Peanut Butter Brussels Sprouts,
  166–167
Pecorino Romano cheese. See
 Parmesan cheese
Pepperoni Rigatoni recipe, 126–127
pine nuts
 Hummus, 178–179
pinto beans
 Breakfast Burritos, 54–55
Plant-Based Caramel Sauce, 217
Plant-Based Creamy Broccoli
 Casserole, 86–87
Plant-Based Parmesan, 212
Plant-Based Protein Waffles, 48–49
Plant-Based Tuscan Alfredo with
 Artichokes & Mushrooms,
 146–147
plant-forward
 about, 8
 getting started, 9–11
popcorn
 Savory Herbaceous, 186
 as a snack, 31
 Sweet Graham Cracker, 187
Portobello Mushroom Burgers with
 Broccoli Slaw, 88–89
potatoes
 Breakfast Burritos, 54–55

Broccoli Cheese Twice-Baked Potatoes, 74–75
Broccoli Potato Hash, 64–65
protein powder
    Blueberry Breakfast Cookies, 37
    Gluten-Free Protein Pancakes, 40–41
Pumpkin Spice Cake, 62–63
Pumpkin Spice Cookies, 192–193
Pumpkin Zucchini Bread, 176–177

Q
quinoa
    Harvest Salad with Maple Vinaigrette, 154–155
    HBE Breakfast Salad, 44–45
    Mushroom & Spinach Enchiladas with Cashew Queso, 94–95
    Quinoa-Stuffed Mushrooms, 184–185
    Stuffed Peppers, 112–113
    Superfood Salad with Lemon Honey Dressing, 152–153
    Sweet Potato Burgers, 84–85
Quinoa-Stuffed Mushrooms, 184–185

R
radishes
    Three-Bean Turkey Chili, 114–115
raisins
    Carrot Cake Cookies, 200–201
reheating prepped meals, 17, 22
Rhatigan, Bailey, story of, 4, 6–7
rice. See also RightRice
    Baked Falafel-Style Balls, 98–99
    HBE Breakfast Salad, 44–45
    Plant-Based Creamy Broccoli Casserole, 86–87
    Roasted Veggie Salad, 158–159
    Veggie Taco Bowls, 67–69
rigatoni. See pasta
RightRice
    about, 29
    Maple Bourbon Salmon with Veggie Rice & Broccoli, 133–135
    Mediterranean Red Pepper Risotto with Shrimp, 138–139
    Mushroom & Spinach Enchiladas with Cashew Queso, 94–95
    Pan-Fried Chicken & Veggies with Rosemary Gravy, 136–137
    Plant-Based Creamy Broccoli Casserole, 86–87
    Teriyaki Salmon Sheet Pan Dinner, 148–149

roasted red peppers
    Fiesta Salad with Plant-Based Ranch, 156–157
    Mediterranean Red Pepper Risotto with Shrimp, 138–139
    Pepperoni Rigatoni, 126–127
    Romesco Dip, 180–181
    Turkey Feta Meatballs with Red Pepper Sauce, 116–117
Roasted Veggie Salad, 158–159
Romesco Dip, 180–181
rosemary
    Pan-Fried Chicken & Veggies with Rosemary Gravy, 136–137

S
salads
    Fiesta Salad with Plant-Based Ranch, 156–157
    Harvest Salad with Maple Vinaigrette, 154–155
    HBE Breakfast Salad, 44–45
    Roasted Veggie Salad, 158–159
    Superfood Salad with Lemon Honey Dressing, 152–153
salmon
    Maple Bourbon Salmon with Veggie Rice & Broccoli, 133–135
    Teriyaki Salmon Sheet Pan Dinner, 148–149
salsa
    about, 29
    Chicken Tacos, 108–109
sauces, adding vegetables to, 10
Savory Herbaceous Popcorn, 186
Savory Nuts, 182–183
seafood. See salmon; shrimp
Shredded BBQ Chicken & Peppers, 120–121
shrimp
    Mediterranean Red Pepper Risotto with Shrimp, 138–139
    Shrimp Cobb Salad, 160–161
Shrimp Cobb Salad, 160–161
snacks, 30–31
Sneaky Turkey Meatloaf, 110–111
So Delicious CocoWhip
    about, 27
    Oatmeal Funfetti Mug Cake, 174–175
soups and stews
    Chipotle Acorn Squash & Kale Stew, 76–77
    vegetables in, 10
sour cream
    Beef Spaghetti Squash with Tzatziki, 128–129

Garlic Dijon Chicken, 101–103
Mushroom Stroganoff, 80–81
Quinoa-Stuffed Mushrooms, 184–185
swap for, 32
spaghetti squash
    Beef Spaghetti Squash with Tzatziki, 128–129
spices, 10–11, 24
spinach
    about, 26
    Artichoke Zucchini Pasta with Roasted Red Pepper Sauce, 96–97
    Bacon & Egg Casserole, 58–59
    Baked Ziti, 106–107
    Beef Spaghetti Squash with Tzatziki, 128–129
    Breakfast Burritos, 54–55
    Fiesta Salad with Plant-Based Ranch, 156–157
    Garlic Dijon Chicken, 101–103
    Harvest Salad with Maple Vinaigrette, 154–155
    HBE Breakfast Salad, 44–45
    Mushroom & Spinach Enchiladas with Cashew Queso, 94–95
    Pan-Fried Chicken & Veggies with Rosemary Gravy, 136–137
    Roasted Veggie Salad, 158–159
    Shredded BBQ Chicken & Peppers, 120–121
    Superfood Salad with Lemon Honey Dressing, 152–153
    Turkey Feta Meatballs with Red Pepper Sauce, 116–117
    Veggie Egg Cups, 38–39
    Veggie Taco Bowls, 67–69
    Zoodles with Artichoke Pesto & Mushrooms, 72–73
stews. See soups and stews
storage containers/bags, 17
storing
    foods, 18–21
    prepped meals, 17
Strawberry Bliss Balls, 169
Stuffed Peppers, 112–113
Sunday Burgers, 142–143
sun-dried tomatoes
    Garlic Dijon Chicken, 101–103
    Superfood Salad with Lemon Honey Dressing, 152–153
    Sweet Graham Cracker Popcorn, 187
    Sweet Potato Burgers, 84–85
    Sweet Potato Fries with Parmesan, 162–163
    Sweet Potato Tacos, 144–145

sweet potatoes
  about, 26
  Broccoli Cheese Twice-Baked
    Potatoes, 74–75
  Broccoli Potato Hash, 64–65
  Cauliflower Curry, 78–79
  Hard-Boiled Egg Plate with
    Roasted Veggies, 50–51
  Harvest Salad with Maple
    Vinaigrette, 154–155
  HBE Breakfast Salad, 44–45
  Loaded Black Bean Quesadillas,
    82–83
  Roasted Veggie Salad, 158–159
  Sweet Potato Burgers, 84–85
  Sweet Potato Fries with
    Parmesan, 162–163
  Sweet Potato Tacos, 144–145

T

tahini
  Beef Spaghetti Squash with
    Tzatziki, 128–129
  Fiesta Salad with Plant-Based
    Ranch, 156–157
  Hummus, 178–179
  Shrimp Cobb Salad, 160–161
  Superfood Salad with Lemon
    Honey Dressing, 152–153
  Turkey Feta Meatballs with Red
    Pepper Sauce, 116–117
Teriyaki Salmon Sheet Pan Dinner,
  148–149
Teriyaki Sauce, 211
Three-Bean Turkey Chili, 114–115
tofu
  Zucchini Lasagna with Plant-
    Based Ricotta, 92–93
tomatoes
  Broccoli Potato Hash, 64–65
  Cashew Queso, 214–215
  Chicken Tacos, 108–109
  Chicken & Veggie Sheet Pan
    Meal, 118–119
  Chipotle Acorn Squash & Kale
    Stew, 76–77
  Garlic Dijon Chicken, 101–103
  Pan-Fried Chicken & Veggies
    with Rosemary Gravy, 136–137
  Plant-Based Tuscan Alfredo with
    Artichokes & Mushrooms,
    146–147
  Romesco Dip, 180–181
  Shrimp Cobb Salad, 160–161
  Sneaky Turkey Meatloaf, 110–111
  Stuffed Peppers, 112–113
  Sunday Burgers, 142–143

Superfood Salad with Lemon
  Honey Dressing, 152–153
Three-Bean Turkey Chili, 114–115
Turkey Veggie Tacos, 130–131
Veggie Taco Bowls, 67–69
tortillas
  Breakfast Burritos, 54–55
  Chicken Sausage Fajitas, 124–125
  Chicken Tacos, 108–109
  Loaded Black Bean Quesadillas,
    82–83
  Mushroom & Spinach Enchiladas
    with Cashew Queso, 94–95
  Sweet Potato Tacos, 144–145
  Turkey Veggie Tacos, 130–131
turkey
  Baked Ziti, 106–107
  Sneaky Turkey Meatloaf, 110–111
  Stuffed Peppers, 112–113
  swap for, 32
  Three-Bean Turkey Chili, 114–115
  Turkey Feta Meatballs with Red
    Pepper Sauce, 116–117
  Turkey Veggie Meatballs, 104–105
  Turkey Veggie Tacos, 130–131
Turkey Feta Meatballs with Red
  Pepper Sauce, 116–117
turkey jerky, as a snack, 31
Turkey Veggie Meatballs, 104–105
Turkey Veggie Tacos, 130–131

V

Vegan Apple Spice Cake, 196–197
Vegan Peanut Butter Cookies,
  202–203
Vegan Vanilla Cupcakes, 189–191
vegetables. *See also specific types*
  about, 25–26
  as snacks, 30
  tips for eating more, 9–10
Veggie Egg Cups, 38–39
veggie rice. *See* RightRice
Veggie Taco Bowls, 67–69

W

walnuts
  Carrot Cake Cookies, 200–201
  Cranberry Almond Granola,
    56–57
  No-Bake Blondies, 194–195
  No-Bake Trail Mix Bars, 172–173
  Peanut Butter Banana Chocolate
    Chip Bars, 198–199
  Pumpkin Zucchini Bread, 176–177
  Sweet Potato Tacos, 144–145
  Zoodles with Artichoke Pesto &
    Mushrooms, 72–73

wine
  Mediterranean Red Pepper
    Risotto with Shrimp, 138–139
  Plant-Based Tuscan Alfredo with
    Artichokes & Mushrooms,
    146–147

Y

yellow squash
  Chicken & Veggie Sheet Pan
    Meal, 118–119
  Pepperoni Rigatoni, 126–127
  Turkey Veggie Tacos, 130–131
yogurt
  about, 27
  Beef Spaghetti Squash with
    Tzatziki, 128–129
  Broccoli Cheese Twice-Baked
    Potatoes, 74–75
  Garlic Dijon Chicken, 101–103
  as a snack, 30
  swaps for, 32
  Veggie Taco Bowls, 67–69

Z

ziti. *See* pasta
Zoodles with Artichoke Pesto &
  Mushrooms, 72–73
zucchini
  about, 26
  Artichoke Zucchini Pasta with
    Roasted Red Pepper Sauce,
    96–97
  Bacon & Egg Casserole, 58–59
  Baked Ziti, 106–107
  Cauliflower Hash, 46–47
  Chicken Sausage Fajitas, 124–125
  Creamy Fettuccine with Avocado,
    90–91
  Fiesta Salad with Plant-Based
    Ranch, 156–157
  HBE Breakfast Salad, 44–45
  Pan-Fried Chicken & Veggies
    with Rosemary Gravy, 136–137
  Pumpkin Zucchini Bread, 176–177
  Sneaky Turkey Meatloaf, 110–111
  Three-Bean Turkey Chili, 114–115
  Turkey Veggie Meatballs, 104–105
  Turkey Veggie Tacos, 130–131
  Veggie Taco Bowls, 67–69
  Zucchini Lasagna with Plant-
    Based Ricotta, 92–93
  Zucchini Parm Boats, 70–71
Zucchini Lasagna with Plant-Based
  Ricotta, 92–93
Zucchini Parm Boats, 70–71